A Clinician's Guide to

Statistics in

Second Edition

A Clinician's Guide to Statistics in Mental Health

Second edition

S. Nassir Ghaemi

Tufts University

Harvard Medical School

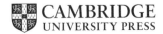

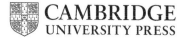

Shaftesbury Road, Cambridge CB2 8EA, United Kingdom

One Liberty Plaza, 20th Floor, New York, NY 10006, USA

477 Williamstown Road, Port Melbourne, VIC 3207, Australia

314–321, 3rd Floor, Plot 3, Splendor Forum, Jasola District Centre,
New Delhi – 110025, India

103 Penang Road, #05–06/07, Visioncrest Commercial, Singapore 238467

Cambridge University Press is part of Cambridge University Press & Assessment,
a department of the University of Cambridge.

We share the University's mission to contribute to society through the pursuit of
education, learning and research at the highest international levels of excellence.

www.cambridge.org
Information on this title: www.cambridge.org/9781108814966

DOI: 10.1017/9781108887526

First published 2009
Second edition 2023

Printed in the United Kingdom by TJ Books Limited, Padstow Cornwall

A catalogue record for this publication is available from the British Library.

Library of Congress Cataloging-in-Publication Data
Names: Ghaemi, S. Nassir, author.
Title: A clinician's guide to statistics in mental health / S. Nassir Ghaemi.
Other titles: A clinician's guide to statistics and epidemiology in mental health | Statistics in mental health
Description: Second edition. | Cambridge, United Kingdom ; New York, NY : Cambridge University Press, 2022. |
Preceded by A clinician's guide to statistics and epidemiology in mental health / S. Nassir Ghaemi. 2009. | Includes
bibliographical references and index.
Identifiers: LCCN 2022033989 (print) | LCCN 2022033990 (ebook) | ISBN 9781108814966 (paperback) | ISBN
9781108887526 (epub)
Subjects: MESH: Psychiatry – methods | Statistics as Topic | Mental Disorders – epidemiology
Classification: LCC RC467.8 (print) | LCC RC467.8 (ebook) | NLM WM 100 |
DDC 616.890072–dc23/eng/20221026
LC record available at https://lccn.loc.gov/2022033989
LC ebook record available at https://lccn.loc.gov/2022033990

ISBN 978-1-108-81496-6 Paperback

In memory of Frederick K. Goodwin, MD

The art of medicine is the art of balancing probabilities.
Adapted from William Osler, 1948, p. 38

Contents

Preface

One of the major problems in the mental health professions is that the majority of clinical researchers in psychiatry are not formally trained in statistics and clinical epidemiology. Imagine if most professors of mathematics were self-educated and never took formal courses in algebra or geometry? Statistics is not something you can pick up on your own, along the way of your busy career as an academic and clinician. It requires time in the classroom – years of time, not months. I know. I had been practicing as a clinical researcher for a decade before I got the opportunity for formal public health training in research methods. After two years of study, I realized how much of my prior research was weak and faulty. That's why I wrote this book: to educate my colleagues, and to try to put into a short work what I had learned in two years. This debate brings out the importance for everyone of better training and education in statistics and research methods. This extra training should be required of those who become researchers in particular. I know that in the 20 years since I had my formal training, many of the changes in my views in psychiatry have had to do with realizing the falsehood of many of the claims about research methods which are used to prop up false clinical judgments, such as the long-term efficacy of antidepressants and anti-psychotics or the debates about the validity of DSM.

In sum, the most prominent "experts" in clinical research methods in academic psychiatry who publish and speak about clinical trial design have never been trained in those topics. My view is that much of the controversy today in psychiatry around statistical issues has to do with the lack of knowledge of the experts. They don't know what they don't know, and yet the field and the pharmaceutical industry relies on their opinions. A new generation is tending to get a few years of post-residency training in schools of public health. That training is a requirement – a necessity, in my opinion – for someone to be a qualified clinical researcher in psychiatry. Meanwhile, the older generation is taking up space with their limited knowledge.

Researchers in psychiatry are uninformed about statistics.

Clinicians fear statistics.

Why?

I'm a clinician. I've treated thousands of patients. I do not have a mathematics degree. I do not have formal statistical training outside a Masters degree in public health. I have been teaching psychiatric residents and medical students about clinical psychiatry for almost three decades, including a course in statistics and evidence-based medicine. I've given many lectures to clinicians. In these settings, one of the most consistent observations I've made is that psychiatric clinicians, whether experienced or early in their training, are afraid of statistics.

I wrote this book to ease their fears but, after a decade in publication, the problem remains. In general, the mere mention of "statistics" in the title of a textbook is a reason for a clinician to avoid it. The question is why.

One possibility is that many clinicians are not highly scientifically oriented. Medicine is a predominantly experiential education, and the science that is involved is mostly of the visual or qualitative kind, such as observing and memorizing the anatomy of the human body. The use of mathematical equations is quite limited.

So, most clinicians in the health professions are wary of mathematics and, therefore, rather allergic to statistics. This matter is not assisted by the fact that most statisticians are the reverse: they are very comfortable with mathematics and, therefore, when they teach statistics they do so with many mathematical equations. Hence, clinicians are turned off by the highly mathematical nature of statistical texts. That is why I tried to write this textbook conceptually, with hardly any mathematics in it.

Preaching about the importance of statistics will not touch the underlying problem, which is an allergy to mathematics. I cannot help this problem. But, I firmly believe, as I say throughout this book, that you cannot be a good clinician unless you have basic statistical knowledge, and it is a sad reality that the vast majority of clinicians and even researchers in psychiatry do not have basic statistical knowledge. This fact produces flawed research and inadequate clinical practice. Many critics of psychiatry and members of the general public go to great lengths to provide complicated reasons for their observation that clinical practice in psychiatry is often inadequate. Besides the complicated reasons brought up in many books, often taken to quite an extreme, there is a very simple one: the lack of knowledge about basic statistical concepts applied to clinical practice.

This book seeks to fill that gap.

This is a book of statistics with no or little requirement for prior experience with it, and with few mathematical equations.

It is written for clinicians and clinical researchers, not statisticians.

I find that clinicians whom I meet in the course of lectures, primarily about psycho-pharmacology, crave this kind of framing of how to read and analyze research studies. Residents and students also are rarely and only minimally exposed to such ideas in training, and, in the course of journal club experiences, I find that they clearly benefit from a systematic exposition of how to assess evidence. Many of the confusing interpretations heard by clinicians are due to their own inability to critically read the literature. They are aware of this fact, but are unable to understand standard statistical texts. They need a book that simply describes what they need to know and is directly relevant to their clinical interests. I could not find such a book to recommend to them.

So, a dozen years ago, I decided to write it.

I now provide a second edition; this has the same basic structure as the first, but with an added section on clinical trials and updated clinical examples, as well as some shortening of technical sections.

Acknowledgments

This book reflects how I have integrated what I learned during the Master of Public Health coursework in the Clinical Effectiveness Program at the Harvard School of Public Health. Before I entered that program in 2002, I had been a psychiatric researcher for almost a decade. When I left that program in 2004, I was completely changed. I had gone into the program thinking I would gain technical knowledge that would help me manipulate numbers, and I did. But, more importantly, I learned how to understand, conceptually, what the numbers meant. As a result, I became a much better researcher, teacher, and peer reviewer, I think. I look back on my pre-MPH days almost as an era of amateur research. My two main teachers in the Clinical Effectiveness program, guides for hundreds of researchers that have gone through their doors for decades, were the epidemiologist Francis Cook and the statistician John Orav.

I would not have been able to take that MPH course of study without the support of a Research Career Development Award (K-23 grant: MH-64189) from the National Institute of Mental Health. Those awards are designed for young researchers and include a teaching component which is meant to advance the formal research skills of the recipient. I hope that this book can be seen in part as the product of taxpayer funds well spent.

Through many lectures, I expressed my enthusiasm to share my new insights about research and statistics, a process of give and take with experienced and intelligent clinicians that led to this book. In the first edition, my friend, the late Jacob Katzow, a clinician in Washington DC, consistently encouraged me to seek to bridge the clinician/researcher divide. The late Frederick K. Goodwin, my closest mentor, was a constant and strong influence on many of the ideas in this book. The first edition benefited from being read by the late Franco Benazzi and from helpful comments from Eric Smith. Richard Marley at Cambridge University Press first suggested this project to me, and Sarah Marsh proposed a second edition and helped see it to conclusion.

Two decades have passed since my first immersion in statistics in psychiatry, and today this field remains, in my opinion, as important as ever.

Why Data Never Speak for Themselves

The beginning of wisdom is to recognize our own ignorance. We mental health clinicians need to start by acknowledging that we are ignorant: we do not know what to do; if we did, we would not need to read anything, much less this book – we could then just treat our patients with the infallible knowledge that we already possess. Although there are dogmatists (and many of them) of this variety – who think that they can be good mental health professionals by simply applying the truths of, say, Freud (or Prozac) to all – this book is addressed to those who know that they do not know, or who at least want to know more.

When faced with persons with mental illnesses, we clinicians need to first determine what their problems are, and then what kinds of treatments to give them. In both cases, in particular the matter of treatment, we need to turn somewhere for guidance: how should we treat patients?

We no longer live in the era of Galen: pointing to the opinions of a wise man is insufficient (though some still do this). Many have accepted that we should turn to science; some kind of empirical research should guide us.

If we accept this view – that science is our guide – then the first question is how are we to understand science?

Science Is Not Simple

This book would be unnecessary if science was simple. I would like to disabuse the reader of any simple notion of science, specifically "positivism": the view that science consists of positive facts, piled one upon another, each of which represents an absolute truth or an independent reality, our business being simply to discover those truths or realities.

This is simply not the case. Science is much more complex.

For the past century scientists and philosophers have debated this matter, and it comes down to this: Facts cannot be separated from theories; science involves deduction, not just induction. In this way, no facts are observed without a preceding hypothesis. Sometimes, the hypothesis is not even fully formulated or even conscious; I may have a number of assumptions that direct me to look at certain facts. It is in this sense that philosophers say that facts are "theory-laden"; between fact and theory, no sharp line can be drawn.

How Statistics Came to Be

A broad outline of how statistics came to be is as follows (Salsburg 2001a): Statistics were developed in the eighteenth century because scientists and mathematicians began to recognize the inherent role of uncertainty in all scientific work. In physics and astronomy, for instance, Pierre-Simon LaPlace realized that certain error was inherent in all calculations.

Instead of ignoring the error, he chose to quantify it, and the field of statistics was born. He even showed that there was a mathematical distribution to the likelihood of errors observed in given experiments. Statistical notions were first explicitly applied to human beings by the nineteenth-century Belgian Lambert Adolphe Quetelet, who applied them to the normal population, and the nineteenth-century French physician Pierre Louis, who applied them to sick persons. In the late nineteenth century, Francis Galton, a founder of genetics and a mathematical leader, applied them to human psychology (studies of intelligence) and worked out the probabilistic nature of statistical inference more fully. His student, Karl Pearson, then took LaPlace one step further and showed that not only is there a probability to the likelihood of error, but even our own measurements are probabilities: "Looking at the data accumulated in biology, Pearson conceived the measurements themselves, rather than errors in the measurement, as having a probability distribution" (Salsburg 2001a, p. 16). Pearson called our observed measurements "parameters" (Greek for "almost measurements"), and he developed staple notions such as the mean and standard deviation. Pearson's revolutionary work laid the basis for modern statistics. But if he was the Marx of statistics (he actually was a socialist), the Lenin of statistics would be the early-twentieth-century geneticist Ronald Fisher, who introduced randomization and p-values, followed by A. Bradford Hill in the mid-twentieth century, who applied these concepts to medical illnesses and founded clinical epidemiology. (The reader will see some of these names repeatedly in the rest of this book; the ideas of these thinkers form the basis of understanding statistics.)

It was Fisher who first coined the term "statistic" (Louis had called it the "numerical method"), by which he meant the observed measurements in an experiment, seen as a reflection of all possible measurements. It is "a number that is derived from the observed measurements and that estimates a parameter of the distribution" (Salsburg 2001a, p. 89). He saw the observed measurement as a random number among the possible measurements that could have been made, and thus "since a statistic is random, it makes no sense to talk about how accurate a single value of it is . . . What is needed is a criterion that depends on the probability distribution of the statistic." How probably valid is the observed measurement, asked Fisher? Statistical tests are all about establishing these probabilities, and statistical concepts are about how we can use mathematical probability to know whether our observations are more or less likely to be correct.

A Scientific Revolution

This process really was a revolution; it was a major change in our thinking about science. Prior to these developments, even the most enlightened thinkers (such as the French Encyclopedists of the eighteenth century, and Auguste Comte in the nineteenth century) saw science as the process of developing absolutely certain knowledge through refinements of sense-observation. Statistics rests on the concept that scientific knowledge, derived from observation using our five senses and aided by technologies, is not absolute. Hence, "the basic idea behind the statistical revolution is that the real things of science are distributions of number, which can then be described by parameters. It is mathematically convenient to embed that concept into probability theory and deal with probability distributions" (Salsburg 2001a, pp. 307–8).

It is thus not an option to avoid statistics if one cares about science. And if one understands science correctly, not as a matter of absolute positive knowledge but as a much more complex probabilistic endeavor (see Chapter 11), then statistics are part and parcel of science.

Some doctors hate statistics, yet they claim to support science. They cannot have it both ways.

A Benefit to Mankind

Statistics thus developed outside of medicine, in other sciences in which researchers realized that uncertainty and error were in the nature of science. Once the wish for absolute truth was jettisoned, statistics would become an essential aspect of all science. And if physics involves uncertainty, how much more uncertainty is there in medicine? Human beings are much more uncertain than atoms and electrons.

The practical results of statistics in medicine are undeniable. If nothing else had been achieved but two things – in the nineteenth century, the end of bleeding, purging, and leeching as a result of Louis' studies; in the twentieth century, the proof of cigarette-smoking -related lung cancer as a result of Hill's studies – we would have to admit that medical statistics have delivered humanity from two powerful scourges.

Numbers Do Not Stand Alone

The history of science shows us that scientific knowledge is not absolute, and that all science involves uncertainty. These truths lead us to a need for statistics. Thus, in learning about statistics, the reader should not expect pure facts; the result of statistical analyses is not unadorned and irrefutable fact; all statistical inference is an act of interpretation, and the result of statistics is more interpretation. This is, in reality, the nature of all science: it is interpretation of facts, not simply facts by themselves.

This statistical reality – the fact that data do not speak for themselves and that therefore positivistic reliance on facts is wrong – is called *confounding bias*. As discussed in the next chapter, observation is fallible: we sometimes think we see what is *not* in fact there. This is especially the case in research on human beings. Consider the assertion that caffeine causes cancer. Numerous studies have shown this; the observation has been made over and over again: among those with cancer, coffee use is high compared to those without cancer. Those are the unadorned facts – and they are wrong. Why? Because coffee drinkers also smoke cigarettes more than non-coffee drinkers. Cigarettes are a confounding factor in this observation, and our lives are chock full of such confounding factors. Meaning: We cannot believe our eyes. Observation is not enough for science; one must try to observe *accurately*, by removing confounding factors. How? In two ways:

1. Experiment, by which we control all other factors in the environment except one, thus knowing that any changes are due to the impact of that one factor. This can be done with animals in a laboratory, but human beings cannot (ethically) be controlled in this way. Enter the randomized clinical trial (RCT) – RCTs are how we experiment with humans to be able to observe accurately.

2. Statistics: Certain methods (like regression modeling; see Chapter 6) have been devised to mathematically correct for the impact of measured confounding factors.

We thus need statistics, either through the design of RCTs or through special analyses, so that we can make our observations accurate and so that we can correctly (and not spuriously) accept or reject our hypotheses.

Science is about hypotheses and hypothesis testing, about confirmation and refutation, about confounding bias and experiment, about randomized clinical trials and statistical analysis: in a word, it is not just about facts. Facts always need to be interpreted. And that is the job of statistics: not to tell us the truth, but to help us get closer to the truth by understanding how to interpret the facts.

Knowing Less, Doing More

That is the goal of this book. If you are a researcher, perhaps this book will explain why you do some of the things you do in your analyses and studies, and how you might improve them. If you are a clinician, hopefully it will put you in a place where you can begin to make independent judgments about studies and not simply be at the mercy of the interpretations of others. It may help you realize that the facts are much more complex than they seem; you may end up "knowing" less than you do now, in the sense that you will realize that much that passes for knowledge is only one among other interpretations. At the same time I hope this statistical wisdom proves liberating: you will be less at the mercy of numbers and more in charge of knowing how to interpret numbers. You will know less but, at the same time, what you do know will be more valid and more solid, and thus you will become a better clinician: applying accurate knowledge rather than speculation, and being more clearly aware of where the region of our knowledge ends and where the realm of our ignorance begins.

Clinical Implications

The founder of modern statistics, Pierre-Simon LaPlace, reportedly said that what we know is much less than what we don't know. This perspective applies to anyone who has decent statistical knowledge and a scientific attitude. Such a person will realize that the application of scientific concepts involves the refutation of hypotheses, not just their confirmation. They will realize that most of our best scientific data refute false beliefs without necessarily replacing them immediately with true beliefs. Hence, as we become more scientific, we realize how many of our ideas were false, and thus we give up beliefs that we used to have. The result is that we will know less, but what we do know will be more solid.

A truly scientifically oriented person must become comfortable with the idea of not knowing many things. Most clinicians believe too strongly that what they think is true. They have a very high threshold for changing their ideas based on scientific evidence, even though they had a very low threshold for accepting those ideas to begin with. This is exactly the opposite of the scientific attitude. A knowledge of statistics is a good vaccine against this kind of common antiscientific attitude, held by many clinicians and even researchers.

2

Why You Cannot Believe Your Eyes

Believe nothing you hear, and only half that you see.

Edgar Allan Poe (Poe 1845)

A core concept in this book is that the validity of any study involves the sequential assessment of Confounding bias, followed by Chance, followed by Causation (what has been called the Three Cs) (Abramson and Abramson 2001).

Any study needs to pass these three hurdles before you should consider accepting its results. Once we accept that no fact or study result is accepted at face value (because no facts can be observed purely, but rather all are interpreted), then we can turn to statistics to see what kinds of methods we should use to analyze those facts. These three steps are widely accepted and form the core of statistics and epidemiology.

The First C: Bias (Confounding)

The first step is bias, by which we mean *systematic* error (as opposed to the random error of chance). Systematic error means that one makes the same mistake over and over again because of some inherent problem with the observations being made. There are subtypes of bias (selection, confounding, measurement), and they are all important, but I will emphasize here what is perhaps the most common and insufficiently appreciated kind of bias: confounding. Confounding has to do with factors, of which we are unaware, that influence our observed results. The concept is best visualized in Figure 2.1.

Hormone Replacement Therapy

As seen in Figure 2.1, the confounding factor is associated with the exposure (or what we think is the cause) and leads to the result. The *real* cause is the confounding factor; the *apparent* cause, which we observe, is just along for the ride. The example of caffeine, cigarettes, and cancer was given in the preceding chapter. Another key example is the case of hormone replacement therapy (HRT). For decades, with much observational experience and large observational studies, most physicians were convinced that HRT had beneficial medical effects in women, especially post-menopausally. Those women who used HRT did better than those who did not use HRT. When finally put to the test in a huge randomized clinical trial (RCT), HRT was found to lead to worse cardiovascular and cancer outcomes than placebo. Why had the observational results been wrong? Because of confounding bias: those women who had used HRT also had better diets and exercised more than women who did not use HRT. Diet and exercise were the confounding factors: they led to better medical outcomes directly, and they were associated with HRT. When the RCT

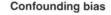

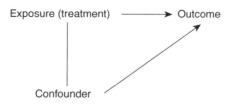

Figure 2.1 Confounding bias

equalized all women who received HRT versus placebo on diet and exercise (as well as all other factors), the direct effect of HRT could finally be observed accurately – and it was harmful to boot (Prentice et al. 2006).

The Eternal Triangle

As one author puts it:

> Confounding is the epidemiologist's eternal triangle. Any time a risk factor, patient charac-teristic, or intervention appears to be causing a disease, side effect, or outcome, the relationship needs to be challenged. Are we seeing cause and effect, or is a confounding factor exerting its unappreciated influence? ... Confounding factors are always lurking, ready to cast doubt on the interpretation of studies.   (Gehlbach 2006, pp. 227–8)

This is the lesson of confounding bias: *We cannot believe our eyes.* Or, perhaps more accurately, we cannot be sure when our observations are right and when they are wrong. Sometimes they are one way or the other, but, more often than not, observation is wrong rather than right due to the high prevalence of confounding factors in the world of medical care.

The kind of confounding bias that led to the HRT debacle had to do with intrinsic characteristics of the population. The doctors had nothing to do with the patients' diets and exercise; the patients themselves controlled those factors. It could turn out that completely independent features, such as hair color or age or gender, are confounding factors in any particular study. These are not controlled by patients or doctors; they are just there in the population and they can affect the results. Two other types of confounding factors exist which are the result of the behavior of patients and doctors: confounding by indication, and measurement bias.

Confounding by Indication

The major confounding factor that results from the behavior of doctors is *confounding by indication* (also called selection bias). This is a classic and extremely poorly appre-ciated source of confusion in medical research. As a clinician, you are trained to be a nonrandomized treater. What this means is that you are taught, through years of supervision and more years of clinical experience, to tailor your treatment decisions to each individual patient. You do not treat patients randomly. You do not say to patient A, take drug X; and to patient B, take drug Y; and to patient C, take drug X; and to patient D, take drug Y – you do not do this without thinking any further about the matter, about why each patient should receive the one drug and not the other. You do not practice randomly; if you did, you should be appropriately sued. However, by practicing nonrandomly, you automatically bias all your experience. You think your patients are doing well because of your treatments, whereas they should be doing well because you are tailoring your treatments *to those who would do well with them*. In other words, it often is not the treatment effects that you are observing, but the treatment effects in specially chosen populations. If you then generalize from those specific patients to the wider population of patients, you will be mistaken.

Measurement Bias: Blinding

I have focused on the first C as confounding bias. The larger topic here is bias, or systematic error, and besides confounding bias there is one other major source of bias: measurement bias (sometimes also called information bias). Here, the issue is not that the outcomes are due to unanalyzed confounding factors, but rather that the outcomes themselves may be inaccurate. The way the outcomes are measured, or the information is obtained on which the outcomes are based, is false. Often this can be related to the impact of either the patients' wishes or the doctors' beliefs; thus, double-blinding is the usual means of handling measurement bias.

Randomization is the best means of addressing confounding bias, and blinding the best means for addressing measurement bias. While blinding is important, it is not as important as randomization. Confounding bias is much more prominent and multivaried than measurement bias. Clinicians often focus on blinding as the means of handling bias; this only addresses the minor part of bias. Unless randomization occurs, or regression modeling or other statistical analyses are conducted, the problem of confounding bias will render study results invalid.

The Second C: Chance

If a study is randomized and blinded successfully, or if observational data are appropriately analyzed with regression or other methods, and there still seems to be a relationship between a treatment and an outcome, we turn to the question of chance. We can then say that this relationship does not seem to be systematically erroneous due to some hidden bias in our observations; now the question is whether it just happened by chance, whether it represents random error.

I will discuss the nature of the hypothesis-testing approach in statistics in more detail in Chapter 8; suffice it to say here that the convention is that a relationship is viewed as being unlikely to be erroneous due to chance if, using mathematical equations designed to measure chance occurrence of associations, it is likely to have occurred 5% of the time, or less frequently, due to chance. This is the famous p-value, which I will discuss more in Chapter 7.

The application of those mathematical equations is a simple matter, and thus the assessment of chance is not complex at all. It is much simpler than assessing bias, but it is correspondingly less important. Usually, it is no big deal to assess chance; bias is the tough part. Yet again, many clinicians equate statistics with p-values and assessing chance. This is one of the least important parts of statistics.

Often what happens is that the first C is ignored, bias is insufficiently examined, and the second C is exaggerated: not just 1, or 2, but 20 or 50 p-values are thrust upon the reader in the course of an article. The p-value is abused until it becomes useless or, worse, misleading.

The problem with chance, usually, is that we focus too much on it, and we misinterpret our statistics. The problem with bias, usually, is we focus too little on it, and we don't even bother with statistics to assess it.

The Third C: Causation

Should a study pass the first two hurdles – bias and chance – it still should not be seen as valid unless we assess it in terms of Causation. This is an even more complex topic, and a part of statistics where clinicians cannot simply look for a number or a p-value to give them an answer. We actually have to use our minds here, and think in terms of ideas, and not simply numbers.

The problem of causation is this: If x is associated with y, and there is no bias or chance error, still we need to then show that x causes y. Not just that Prozac *is associated with* less depression, but that Prozac *causes* less depression. How can we do this? A p-value will not do it for us.

This is a problem that has been central to the field of clinical epidemiology for decades. The classic handling of it has been ascribed to the work of the great medical epidemiologist A. Bradford Hill, who was central to the research on tobacco and lung cancer. A major problem with that research was that randomized studies could not be done: You smoke, you don't, and see me in 40 years to see who has cancer. This could not practically or ethically be done. This research was observational and liable to bias; Hill and others devised methods to assess bias, but they always had the problem of never being able to completely remove doubt. The cigarette companies, of course, exploited this matter to constantly magnify this doubt and delay the inevitable day when they would be forced to back off from their dangerous business.

With all this observational research, they would argue to Hill and his colleagues, you still cannot prove that cigarettes *cause* lung cancer. And they were right. So Hill set about trying to clarify how one might prove that something causes anything in medical research with human beings.

I Hill basically pointed out that causation cannot be derived from any one source; rather, it could be inferred by an accumulation of evidence from multiple sources (see chapter 14).

It is not enough to say a study is valid; one also wants to know if these results are replicated by multiple studies, if they are supported by biological studies in animals on mechanisms of effect, if they follow certain patterns consistent with causation (like a dose-response relationship), and so on.

For our purposes, we might at least insist on replication. No single study should stand on its own, no matter how well done. Even after crossing the barriers of bias and chance, we should ask of a study that it be replicated and confirmed in other samples and other settings.

Most clinicians and researchers pay too much attention to blinding and too little attention to confounding bias. Routinely, when I ask residents or clinicians what is the key reason for doing randomized trials, they reply blinding. They do not understand that randomization is more important than blinding, for the reasons given earlier. Blinding, in fact, doesn't matter if there is no randomization. All blinding does is affect the psychological expectancy of human beings in clinical trials. But psychological expectancy is only one bias factor out of many. The many additional factors include natural history, severity of illness, and multiple other biological factors which are not controlled in a study unless randomization occurs. They far outweigh psychological expectancy in their effects of producing bias. Clinicians and researchers simply do not understand the rationale for randomization because they do not appreciate the concept of confounding bias. The concept of confounding bias is the most important concept in statistics for both clinical practice and clinical research.

Confounding bias, chance, and causation: these are the three basic notions that underlie statistics and epidemiology. If clinicians understand these three concepts, then they will know that they will be able to believe their eyes more validly.

Levels of Evidence

The term "evidence" has become about as controversial as the word "unconscious" had been in the Freudian heyday, or as the term "proletariat" was in another arena. It means many things to many people, and, for some, it elicits reverent awe – or reflexive aversion. This is because, like the other terms, it is linked to a movement – in this case evidence-based medicine (EBM) – which is currently quite influential and, with this influence, has attracted both supporters and critics.

This book is not about EBM per se, nor is it simply an application of EBM, although it is, in my view, consistent with EBM, rightly understood. I will expand on that topic further in Chapter 12, but for now I would like to emphasize at the very start what I take to be the most important feature of EBM: the concept of *levels of evidence.*

Origins of EBM

It may be worthwhile to note that the originators of the EBM movement in Canada (such as David Sackett) toyed with different names for what they wanted to do; they initially thought about the phrase "science-based medicine" but opted for the term "evidence" instead. This is perhaps unfortunate since science tends to engender respect, while evidence seems a vaguer concept. Hence, we often see proponents of EBM (mistakenly, in my view) saying things like "That opinion is not evidence-based" or "Those articles are not evidence-based." The folly of this kind of language is evident if we use the term in science instead: "That opinion is not science-based" or "Those articles are not science-based." Once we use the term "science," it becomes clear that such statements beg the question of what science means. Most of us would be open to such a discussion (which I touched on in the Introduction). Yet (ironically, perhaps, due to the success of the EBM movement) many use the term "evidence" without pausing to think what it means. If some study is not "evidence-based," then what is it? "Nonevidence" based? "Opinion" based. But is there such a thing as "nonevidence"? Is there no opinion in evidence? Stated otherwise, do the facts speak for themselves? We have seen that they do not, which tells us that those who say things such as "That study is not evidence-based" are basically revealing their positivism: they could just as well say "That study is not science-based" because they have a very specific meaning in mind for science, which is in fact positivism. Since positivism is false, this extreme and confused notion of evidence is also false.

There is no inherent opposition between evidence and opinion, because "evidence," if meant to be "facts," always involves interpretation (which involves opinions or subjective assessments), as we discussed earlier.

In other words, all opinions are types of evidence; any perspective at all is based on some kind of evidence: thus, there is no such thing as "nonevidence."

In my reading of EBM, the basic idea is that we need to understand what kinds of evidence we use, and we need to use the best kinds we can: this is the concept of *levels* of evidence. EBM is *not* about an opposition between having evidence or not having evidence; it is about ranking different kinds of evidence (since we always have some kind of evidence or another).

Specific Levels of Evidence

The EBM literature has various definitions of specific levels of evidence. The main EBM text uses letters (A through D). I prefer numbers (1 through 5), and I think the specific content of the levels should vary depending on the field of study. The basic constant idea is that randomized studies are higher levels of evidence than nonrandomized studies, and that the lowest level of evidence consists of case reports, expert opinion, or the consensus of the opinion of clinicians or investigators.

Levels of evidence provide clinicians and researchers with a roadmap that allows consistent and justified comparison of different studies so as to adequately compare and contrast their findings. Various disciplines have applied the concept of levels of evidence in slightly different ways, and in psychiatry no consensus definition exists. In my view, in mental health, the following five levels of evidence best apply (Table 3.1), ranked from level I as the highest and level V as the lowest.

The key feature to keep in mind with regard to levels of evidence is that each level has its own strengths and weaknesses and, as a result, no single level is completely useful or completely useless. All other things being equal, however, as one moves from level V to level I, increasing rigor and probable scientific accuracy occurs.

Level V means a case report or a case series (a few case reports strung together), or an expert's opinion, or the consensus of experts or clinicians or investigators opinions (such as in treatment algorithms), or the personal clinical experience of clinicians, or the words of wisdom of Great Professors (like Freud or Kraepelin or Galen or Marx or Adam Smith). All of this is the same level of evidence: the lowest. This does not mean that such evidence is wrong, nor does it mean that it is *not* evidence; it is a *kind* of evidence, just a weak kind. It

Table 3.1 Levels of evidence

Level I: Double-blind randomized trials
Ia: Placebo-controlled monotherapy
Ib: Non placebo-controlled comparison trials, or placebo-controlled add-on therapy trials
Level II: Open randomized trials
Level III: Observational studies
IIIa: Nonrandomized, controlled studies
IIIb: Large nonrandomized, uncontrolled studies (n>100)
IIIc: Medium-sized nonrandomized, uncontrolled studies (100 > n > 50)
Level IV: Small observational studies (nonrandomized, uncontrolled, 50 > n > 10)
Level V: Case series (n < 10), Case report (n = 1), Expert opinion

could turn out that a case report is correct, and a randomized study wrong but, in general, randomized studies are much more likely to be correct than case reports. We simply cannot know when a case report, or an expert opinion, or a saying of Freud or Marx, is right and when it is wrong. More often than not, such cases or opinions are wrong rather than right, but this does not mean that any single case or opinion might not, in fact, be correct. Authority is not, as with Rome, the last word.

All of medicine functioned on level V until the revolutionary work of Pierre Louis, whose numerical method introduced level IV: the small observational study. How small is small? This will vary based on the topic of study, but one approach might be to say that a moderate effect size in clinical psychiatry requires two groups with samples of about 25 each for detection with p-values; hence, a sample smaller than 50 might be considered "small"; for other disciplines and other outcomes, different numbers might be considered small. For instance, in clinical genetics, thousands of patients are required to detect the generally small genetic effect sizes being measured – thus, 100 might be considered a small sample in that field.

Observational studies are not randomized, and are open-label. Level III is the large observational study, such as the cohort study – the staple of the field of epidemiology. Here we would place such large and highly informative studies as the Framingham Heart Study, the Nurses Health Study, and so on. In those cases, the large samples involve more than 1,000 patients. One might say in psychiatry that even greater than 50–100 might be considered large depending on the effect sizes being measured. Such observational studies (in this level as well as level IV) can be prospective or retrospective, with prospective studies being considered more valid (thus one might label them IIIa as opposed to IIIb for retrospective studies) due to the a priori specification of outcomes as well as the usual careful rating and assessment of outcomes (as opposed to retrospective assessment of outcomes, as is commonly the case in chart reviews, for instance).

Levels II and I take us to the highest levels of evidence due to randomization, which, as we saw, is the best tool to minimize or remove confounding bias. Level II represents open (not double-blind) randomized clinical trials (RCTs) and level I represents double-blind RCTs. Within each level one might subgroup for small studies (in psychiatry < 50 subjects; IIb or Ic) versus large studies (>50 subjects; IIa or Ib), and within level I studies, we might also subgroup based on use of placebo in large studies (Ia, the highest level of evidence).

Judging between Conflicting Evidence

The recognition of levels of evidence allows one to have a guiding principle by which to assess a literature. Basic rules are:

1. All other things being equal, a study at a higher level of evidence provides more valid (or powerful) results than one at a lower level.
2. Base judgments as much as possible on the highest levels of evidence.
3. Levels II and III are often the highest level of evidence attainable for complex conditions, and are to be valued in those circumstances.
4. Higher levels of evidence do not guarantee certainty; any one study can be wrong, thus look for replicability.
5. Within any level of evidence, studies may conflict based on other methodological issues not captured by the parameters used to provide the general outlines of levels of evidence.

One major advantage of a levels-of-evidence approach to an examination of data is that there is not a huge leap between double-blind, placebo-controlled studies and other, less rigorous levels. In other words, clinicians and some academics sometimes imagine that all studies that are not level I, double-blind RCTs are equivalent in terms of rigor, accuracy, reliability, and information. In reality, there are many intermediate levels of evidence, each with particular strengths as well as limits. Open randomized studies and large observational studies, in particular, can be extremely informative and sometimes as accurate as level I studies. The concept of levels of evidence can also help clinicians who are loath to rely on level I controlled clinical trials, especially if those results contradict their own level V clinical experiences. While the advantages to level V data mainly revolve around hypothesis generation, to devalue higher levels of evidence is unscientific and dangerous.

In my view, the concept of levels of evidence is the key concept of EBM. With it, EBM is valuable; without it, EBM is misunderstood.

Bias

What the doctor saw with one, two, or three patients may be both acutely noted and accurately recorded; but what he saw is not necessarily related to what he did.
(Austin Bradford Hill) (Hill, 1962, p. 4)

The issue of bias is so important that it deserves even more clarification than the discussion I gave in Chapter 2. In this chapter, I will examine the two basic types of bias: confounding bias and measurement bias.

Confounding Bias

To restate, the basic notion of confounding bias was shown in Figure 2.1, the "eternal triangle" of the epidemiologist.

The idea is that we cannot believe our eyes, that, in the course of observation, other factors of which we may not be aware (confounding factors) could be influencing our results. The associations we think are happening (between treatment and outcome, or exposure and result) may be due to something else altogether. We have to constantly be skeptical about what we think we see; we have to be aware of, and even expect, that what seems to be happening is not really happening at all. The truth lies below the surface of what is observed: the "facts" cannot be taken at face value.

Put in epidemiological language: "Confounding in its ultimate essence is a problem with a particular estimate – a question of whether the magnitude of the estimate at hand could be *explained* in terms of some *extraneous* factor." And again: "By 'extraneous factor' is meant something other than the exposure or the illness – a characteristic of the study subjects or of the process of securing information on them" (Miettinen and Cook 1981, p. 600).

Confounding bias is handled either by *preventing* it, through randomization in *study design*, or by *removing* it, through regression models in *data analysis*. Neither option is guaranteed to remove all confounding bias from a study, but randomization is much closer to being definitive than regression (or any other statistical analysis; see Chapter 5): one can better prevent confounding bias than remove it after the fact.

Another way of understanding the cardinal importance of confounding bias is to recognize that all medical research is about getting at the truth about some topic, and to do so one has to make an unbiased assessment of the matter at hand. This is the basic idea that underlies what A. Bradford Hill called "the philosophy of the clinical trial." Here is how this founder of modern epidemiology explained the matter:

> The reactions of human beings to most diseases are, under any circumstances, extremely variable. They do not all behave uniformly and decisively. They vary, and that is where the

trouble begins. "What the doctor saw" with one, two, or three patients may be both acutely noted and accurately recorded; but *what he saw is not necessarily related to what he did*. The assumption that it is so related, with a handful of patients, perhaps mostly recovering, perhaps mostly dying, must, not infrequently, give credit where no credit is due, or condemn when condemnation is unjust. The field of medical observation, it is necessary to remember, is often narrow in the sense that no one doctor will treat many cases in a short space of time; it is wide in the sense that a great many doctors may each treat a few cases. Thus, with a somewhat ready assumption of cause and effect, and, equally, a neglect of the laws of chance, the literature becomes filled with conflicting cries and claims, assertions and counterassertions. It is thus, for want of an adequately controlled test, that various forms of treatment have, in the past, become unjustifiably, even sometimes harmfully, established in everyday medical practice ... It is this belief, or perhaps state of unbelief, that has led in the last few years to a wider development in therapeutics of the more deliberately experimental approach.   (Hill 1962a, pp. 3–4 [italics added])

Hill is referring to bloodletting and all that Galenic harm that doctors had practiced since Christ walked the earth. It is worth emphasizing that those who cared about statistics in medicine were interested as much, if not more, in disproving what doctors actually *do*, rather than proving what doctors *should* do. We cause a lot of harm as clinicians; we always have and we likely still are. The main reason for this morally compelling fact is this phenomenon of confounding bias. We know not what we do, yet we think we know.

This is the key implication of confounding bias: that we think we know things are such-and-such, but in fact they are not. This might be called *positive* confounding bias: the idea that there is a fact (drug X improves disease Y) when in fact that fact is wrong. But there is also another kind of confounding bias: it may be that we think certain facts do not exist (say, a drug does not cause problem Z), when in fact that fact does exist (the drug does cause problem Z). We may not be aware of the fact because of confounding factors which hide the true relationship between drug X and problem Z from our observation: this is called *negative* confounding bias.

We live in a confounded world: we never really know whether what we are observing actually is happening as it seems, or whether what we fail to observe might actually be happening.

Let us see two examples of how these cases play out in clinical practice.

Effect Modification

An important concept to distinguish from confounding bias is effect modification (EM). Effect modification is related to confounding in that in both cases the relationship between the exposure (or treatment) and the outcome is affected. The difference is conceptual. In confounding bias, the exposure really has no relation to the outcome at all; it is only through the confounding factor that any relation exists. Another way of putting this is that in confounding bias, the confounding factor causes the outcome; the exposure does not cause the outcome at all. The confounding factor is not on the causal pathway of exposure and outcome. In other words, it is not the case that the exposure causes the outcome through the mediation of the confounding factor; the confounding factor is not merely a mechanism whereby the exposure causes the outcome. To repeat a classic example, numerous epidemiological studies find an association between coffee drinking and cancer, but this is due to the confounding effect of cigarette smoking: more coffee drinkers smoke cigarettes, and it is the

Example 1 Confounding by indication: Antidepressant discontinuation in bipolar depression

Confounding by indication (also called selection bias) is the type of confounding bias of which clinicians may be aware, though it is important to point out that confounding bias is not just limited to clinicians selecting patients nonrandomly for treatment. There can also be other factors that influence outcomes, of which clinicians are entirely unaware or which clinicians do not influence at all (e.g., patients' dietary or exercise habits, gender, race, socioeconomic status). Confounding by indication, though, refers to the fact that, as mentioned in Chapter 2, *clinicians practice medicine nonrandomly*. We do not haphazardly (one hopes) give treatments to patients; we seek to treat some patients with some drugs, and other patients with other drugs, based on judgments about various predictive factors (age, gender, type of illness, kinds of current symptoms, past side effects) that we think will maximize the chances that the patient will respond to the treatments we provide. The better we are in this process, the better our patients do and the better clinicians we are. However, being a good clinician means that we will be bad researchers. If we conclude from our clinical successes that the treatments we use are quite effective, we may be mistaking the potency of our pills for our own clinical skills. Good outcomes simply mean that we know how to match patients to treatments; it does not mean that the treatments, in themselves or in general, are effective. To really know what the treatments do, we need to disentangle what we do as clinicians from what the pills do as chemicals.

An example of likely confounding by indication from the psychiatric literature follows: An observational study of antidepressant discontinuation in bipolar disorder (Altshuler et al. 2003) found that after initial response to a mood stabilizer plus an antidepressant, those who stayed on the combination stayed well longer than those in whom the antidepressant was stopped. In other words, at face value the study seems to show that long-term continuation of antidepressants in bipolar disorder appears to lead to better outcomes. This study was published in the *American Journal of Psychiatry* (*AJP*) without any further statistical analysis, and this apparent result was discussed frequently at conferences for years subsequent to its publication.

But the study does not pass the first test of the Three Cs. The first question, and one never asked by the peer reviewers of *AJP* (see Chapter 17 for a discussion of peer review), is whether there might be any confounding bias in this observational study.

Readers should begin to assess this issue by putting themselves in the place of the treating clinicians. Why would one stop antidepressant after acute recovery? There is a literature that suggests that antidepressants can cause or worsen rapid cycling in patients with bipolar disorder. So, if a patient has rapid-cycling illness, some clinicians would be inclined to stop the antidepressant after acute recovery. If a patient had a history of antidepressant-induced mania that was common or severe, some clinicians might not continue the antidepressant. Perhaps if the patient had bipolar disorder type I, some clinicians would be less likely to continue antidepressants than if the patient had bipolar disorder type II. These are issues of selection bias, or so-called confounding by indication: the doctor decides what to do nonrandomly. Another way to frame the issue is this: we don't know how many patients did worse because they were taken off antidepressants versus how many were taken off because they were doing worse. There may also be other confounders that just happen to be the case: there may be more males in one group, a younger age of onset in one group, or a greater severity of illness in one group. To focus only on the potential confounding factor of rapid cycling, if the group in whom antidepressants were stopped had more rapid cyclers (due to confounding by indication) than the other group (in whom antidepressant use was continued), then the observed finding that the antidepressant discontinuation group relapsed earlier than the other group would be due to the natural history of rapid-cycling illness: rapid cyclers relapse more rapidly than nonrapid cyclers. This would then be a classic case of confounding bias, and the results would have nothing to do with the antidepressants.

It may not be, in fact, that any of these potential confounders actually influenced the results of the study. However, the researchers and readers of the literature should think about and examine such possibilities. The authors of such studies usually do so in an initial table of demographic and clinical characteristics (often referred to as "Table 1" because it is needed in practically every clinical study; see Chapter 5). The first table should generally be a comparison of clinical and demographic variables in the groups being studied to see if there are any differences which might be confounders. For instance, if 50% of the anti-depressant continuation group had rapid cycling and so did 50% of the discontinuation group, then such confounding effects would be unlikely because both groups are equally exposed. The whole point of randomized studies is that randomization more or less guarantees that all variables will be 50–50 distributed *across* groups (the key point is equal representation *across* groups, no matter what the absolute value of each variable is *within* each group: i.e., 5% vs 50% vs 95%). In an observational study, one needs to look at each variable one by one. If such possible confounders are identified, the authors then have two potential solutions: stratification or regression models (see Appendix).

It is worth emphasizing that the baseline assessment of potential confounders in two groups has nothing to do with p-values. A common mistake is for researchers to compare two groups, note a p-value above 0.05, and conclude that there is "no difference" and thus no confounding effect. However, such use of p-values is generally thought to be inappropriate, as will be discussed further, because such comparisons are usually not the primary purpose of the study (the study might be focused on antidepressant outcome, not age or gender differences between groups). In addition, such studies are underpowered to detect many clinical and demographic differences (that is, they have an unacceptably high possibility of a false negative or type II error), and thus p-value comparisons are irrelevant.

Perhaps the most important reason that p-values are irrelevant here is that any notable difference, even if not statistically significant, in a confounding factor (e.g., severity of illness) may have a major impact on an apparently statistically significant result with the experimental variable (e.g., antidepressant efficacy). Such a confounding effect may be big enough to completely swamp, or at least lessen the difference on the experimental variable such that a previously statistically significant (but small to moderate in effect size) result is no longer statistically significant. How large can such confounding effects be? The general rule of 10% or larger, *irrespective of statistical significance*, seems to hold (see Chapter 5). The major concern is not whether there is a statistically significant difference in a potential confounder, but rather whether there is a difference big enough to cause concern that our primary results may be distorted.

Example 2 Negative confounding: Substance abuse and antidepressant-associated mania

The possibility of negative confounding bias is often underappreciated. If one only looks at each variable in a study, one by one (univariate), compared to an outcome, each one of them might be unassociated; but if one puts them all into a regression model, so that confounding effects between the variables are controlled, then some of them might turn out to be associated with the outcome (see Appendix).

Here is an example from our research on the topic of substance abuse as a predictor of antidepressant-related mania (ADM) in bipolar disorder. In the previous literature, one study had found such an association with a direct univariate comparison of substance abuse and the outcome of ADM (Goldberg and Whiteside 2002). No regression modeling was conducted. We decided to try to replicate this study in a new sample of 98 patients, using regression models to adjust for confounding factors (Manwani et al. 2006). In our initial analysis, with a simple univariate comparison of substance abuse and ADM, we found no link at all: ADM occurred in 20.7% of substance abuse subjects and 21.4% of non-substance abuse subjects. The relative risk was almost exactly the null value, with confidence intervals (CIs) symmetrical about the null (RR = 0.97, 95% CIs 0.64, 1.48). There was just no effect at all. If we had reported our result analyzed exactly as the previous study, the scientific literature would have existed of two identically designed conflicting results. This is quite common in observational studies, which are rife with confounding bias in all directions. Our study would have been publishable at that step, like so many others, and it would have just added one more confounded result to the psychiatric literature. However, after we conducted a multivariate regression, and thereby adjusted the effect of substance abuse for multiple other variables, not only did we observe a relationship between substance abuse and ADM, it was a an effect size of about a three-fold increased risk (OR = 3.09, 95% CIs [0.92, 10.40]). The wide CIs did not allow us to rule out the null hypothesis with 95% certainty, but they were definitely skewed in the direction of a highly probable positive effect.

cigarettes, completely and entirely, that cause the cancer; coffee itself has not increased the cancer risk. This is confounding bias.

Let us suppose that the risk of cancer is higher in women smokers than in men smokers; this is no longer confounding bias, but EM. There is some interaction between gender and cigarette smoking, such that women are more prone biologically to the harmful effects of cigarettes (this is a hypothetical example). But we have no reason to believe that being female per se leads to cancer, as opposed to being male. Gender itself does not cause cancer: it is not a confounding factor, it merely modifies the risk of cancer with the exposure, cigarette smoking.

We might then contrast the differences between confounding bias and EM by comparing Figure 2.1 with Figure 4.1.

When a variable affects the relationship between exposure and outcome, then a conceptual assessment needs to be made about whether the third variable directly causes the outcome but is not caused by the exposure (then it is a confounding factor), or whether the third variable does not cause the exposure and seems to modify the exposure's effects (then it is an effect modifier). In either case, those other variables are important to assess so that we can get a more valid understanding of the relationship between the exposures of interest and outcomes. Put another way, there is no way that a simple one-to-one comparison (as in univariate analyses) gives us a valid picture of what is really happening in observational experience. Both confounding bias and effect modification occur a lot, and they need to be assessed in statistical analyses.

Measurement Bias

The other major type of bias, less important than confounding, is measurement bias. Here the issue is whether the investigator or the subject measures, or assesses, the outcome

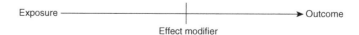
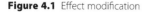

Figure 4.1 Effect modification

validly. The basic idea is that in subjective outcomes (like pain), the subject or investigator might be biased in favor of what is being studied. In more objective outcomes (like mortality), this bias will be less likely. Blinding (single – of the subject; double – of the subject and investigator) is used to minimize this bias.

Many clinicians mistake blinding for randomization. It is not uncommon for authors to write about "blinded studies" without informing us whether the study was randomized or not. In practice, blinding always happens with randomization (it is impossible to have a double-blind but then nonrandomly decide about treatments to be given). However, it does not work the other way around. One can randomize and not blind a study (open randomized studies), and this can be legitimate. Thus, blinding is optional; it can be present or not, depending on the study; but randomization is essential: it is what marks out the least-biased kind of study.

If one has a "hard" outcome, like death or stroke, where patients and subjects really cannot influence the outcomes based on their subjective opinions, blinding is not a key feature of RCTs. On the other hand, most psychiatric studies have "soft" outcomes, like changes on symptom rating scales, and in such settings blinding is important.

Just like one needs to show that randomization is *successful* (see next chapter), one ought to show that blinding has been successful during a study. This would entail assessments by investigators and subjects of their best guess (usually at the end of a study) regarding which treatment (e.g., drug vs placebo) was received. If the guesses are random, then one can conclude that blinding was successful; if the guesses correlate with the actual treatments given, then potential measurement bias can be present.

This matter is rarely studied. In one example, a double-blind study of alprazolam versus placebo for anxiety disorder, researchers assessed 129 patients and investigators about the allocated treatment after 8 weeks of treatment (Basoglu et al. 1997). The investigators guessed alprazolam correctly in 82% of cases and they guessed placebo correctly in 78% of cases. Patients guessed correctly in 73% and 70% of cases, respectively. The main predictor of correct guessing was presence of side effects. Treatment response did not predict correct guessing of blinded treatment.

If this study is correct, blinded studies really reflect about 20–30% blinding; otherwise, patients and researchers make correct estimations and may bias results, at least to some extent. This unblinding effect may be strongest with drugs that have notable side effects.

An example might be found in randomized studies of quetiapine for acute bipolar depression (which led to a Food and Drug Administration [FDA] indication). That drug was found effective in doses of 300 mg/d or higher, which produced sedation in about one-half of patients given quetiapine (Calabrese et al. 2005). Given the much higher rate of sedation with this drug than placebo, the question can legitimately be asked whether this study was at best only partially blinded.

Measurement bias also comes into play in *not* noticing side effects. For instance, when serotonin reuptake inhibitors (SRIs) were first developed, early clinical trials did not have rating scales for sexual function. Since that side effect was not measured explicitly, it was underreported (people were reluctant to discuss sex). Observational experience identified much more sexual dysfunction than had been mistakenly reported in the early RCTs, and this clinical experience was confirmed by later RCTs that used specific sexual function rating scales.

Measurement bias is also sometimes called misclassification bias, especially in observational studies, when outcomes are inaccurately assessed. For instance, it may be that we conduct a chart review of whether antidepressants cause mania, but we had assessed manic symptoms unsystematically (e.g., rating scales for mania are not used usually in clinical practice), and then we recorded those assessments poorly (the charts might be messy, with brief notes rather than extensive descriptions). With such material, it is likely that at least mild hypomanic or manic episodes would be missed and reported as not existing. The extent of such misclassification bias can be hard to determine.

Chapter 5

Randomization

The most effective way to solve the problem of confounding is by the study design method of *randomization*. This is simply stated, but I would venture to say that this simple statement is the most revolutionary and profound discovery of modern medicine. I would include all the rest of medicine's discoveries in the past century – penicillin, heart transplants, kidney transplants, immunosuppression, gene therapies, all of it – and I would say that all of these specific discoveries are less important than the general idea, the revolutionary idea, of randomization; this is so because without randomization, most of the rest of medicine's discoveries would not have been discovered: it is the power of randomization that allows us, usually, to differentiate the true from the false, a real breakthrough from a false claim.

Counting

I previously mentioned that medical statistics was founded on the groundbreaking study of Pierre Louis, in Paris of the 1840s, when he counted about 40 patients and showed that those with pneumonia who received bleeding died sooner than those who did not. Some basic facts – like the fallacy of bleeding, or the benefits of penicillin – can be established easily enough by just counting some patients. But most medical effects are not as huge as the harm of bleeding or the efficacy of penicillin. We call those "large effect sizes": with just 40 patients one can easily show the benefit or the harm. Most medical effects, though, are smaller: they are medium or small effect sizes, and thus they can get lost in the "noise" of confounding bias. Other factors in the world can either obscure those real effects or make them appear to be present when they are not.

How can we separate real effects from the noise of confounding bias? This is the question that randomization answers.

The First RCT: The Kuala Lumpur Insane Asylum Study

A historical pause may be useful here. Ronald Fisher is usually credited with originating the concept of randomization. Fisher did so in the setting of agricultural studies in the 1920s: certain fields randomly received a certain kind of seed, others fields received other seeds. A. Bradford Hill is credited with adapting the concept to the first human randomized clinical trial (RCT): a study of streptomycin for pneumonia in 1948. Multiple RCTs in other conditions followed right away in the 1950s, the first in psychiatry involving lithium in 1952, and then the antipsychotic chlorpromazine in 1954. This is the standard history, and it is correct in the sense that Fisher and Hill were clearly the first to formally develop the concept of randomization and to recognize its conceptual importance for statistics and science. But there is a hidden history, one that is directly relevant to the mental health professions.

As a historical matter, the first application of randomization in any scientific study appears to have been published by the American philosopher and physicist Charles Sanders Peirce in the late 1860s (Stigler 1986). Peirce did not seem to follow up on his innovation, however. Decades passed, and as statistical concepts began to seep into medical consciousness, it seems that the notion of randomization also began to come into being.

In 1905, in the main insane asylum of Kuala Lumpur, Malaysia, the physician William Fletcher decided to do an experiment to test his belief that white rice was *not*, as some claimed, the source of beriberi (Fletcher 1907). He chose to do the study in the insane asylum because patients' diets and environment could be fully controlled there. He obtained the permission of the government (though not the patients), and assigned consecutive patients to receive either white or brown rice. For one year, the two groups received identical diets except for the different types of rice. Fletcher had conducted the first RCT, and it occurred in psychiatric patients, in an assessment of diet (not drug treatment). Further, the result of the RCT refuted, rather than confirmed, the investigator's hypothesis: Fletcher found that beriberi happened in 24/120 (20%) who received white rice, versus only 2/123 (1.6%) who received brown rice; 18/120 (15%) on the white rice diet died of beriberi, versus none on the brown rice diet (Silverman 1998). Fisher had not invented p-values yet, but if Fletcher had access to them, he would have seen that the chance likelihood of his findings was less than 1 in 1,000 ($p < 0.0001$); as it was, Fletcher knew that the difference between 20% and 2% was large enough to matter.

Arguably, Fletcher had stumbled on the most powerful method of modern medical research. Since not all who ate white rice developed beriberi, the absolute effect size was not large enough to make it an obvious connection. But, using modern terms and methods, the risk ratio (RR), which is a type of what is now called relative risk (the other type being the odds ratio), was indeed quite large (applying modern methods, the RR was 12.3, which is slightly larger than the association of cigarette smoking and lung cancer; the 95% confidence intervals are 3.0 to 50.9, indicating almost total certitude of a three-fold or larger effect size). It took randomization to clear out the noise and let the real effect be seen. At the same time, Fletcher had also discovered the method's premier capacity: its ability to disabuse us of our mistaken clinical observations.

Randomizing Liberals and Conservatives, Blondes and Brunettes

How do we engage in randomization?

We do it by randomly assigning patients to a treatment versus a control (like placebo, or another treatment). You get drug, you get placebo, you get drug, you get placebo, and so on. By doing so randomly, after a large enough number of persons, we ensure that the two groups – drug and placebo – are equal in *all* factors except the experimental choice of receiving drug or placebo. There will be equal numbers of males and females in both groups, equal numbers of old and young persons, equal numbers of those with more severe illness and less severe illness – all the *known* potential confounding factors will be equal in both groups, and thus there will be no *differential* biasing effect of those factors on the results. But more: suppose it turns out in a century that hair color affects our results, or political affiliation, or something apparently ridiculous like how one puts on one's pants in the morning; still, there will be equal numbers of blonds and brunettes in both groups, and equal numbers of liberal and conservatives (we won't prejudge which group would have a worse outcome), and equal numbers of those who put their pants on left leg first versus right leg first in both groups. In other words, all the *unknown* potential confounding factors would also be equalized between both groups.

This is the power of randomization: *all* potential confounding factors – *known or unknown* – should be equalized between the groups, such that the results should be valid, *at face value, now and forever.* (One is tempted to add "Amen," which would be the chorus for proponents of ivory-tower EBM; see Chapter 12.)

This is obviously the ideal situation; RCTs can be invalid, or less valid, due to multiple other design factors outside of randomization (see next chapter). But, if all other aspects of an RCT are well-designed, the impact of randomization is that it can provide something as close to absolute truth as is possible in the world of medical science.

Measuring Success of Randomization

All these claims are contingent on the RCT being well-designed. And the first matter of importance is that the randomization needs to be "successful," by which we mean that, as best as we can tell, the two groups are in fact equal on almost all variables that we can measure. Usually this is assessed in a table (usually the first table in a paper, and thus often referred to as "Table One") comparing clinical and demographic characteristics of the two (or more) randomized subgroups in the overall sample.

The most important feature that differentiates whether randomization will be successful is *sample size*. This is by far the most important factor, and it is easy to understand. Even before randomization as a concept was developed, the relevance of sample size for confounding bias was identified by a nineteenth-century founder of statistics, Quetelet, who wrote in 1835: "The greater the number of individuals observed, the more do individual peculiarities, whether physical or moral, become effaced, and allow the general facts to predominate, by which society exists and is preserved" (quoted in Stigler 1986, p. 172).

If I flip a coin twice, it might turn out heads–heads, or tails–tails, rather frequently; I have to flip it lots of times for it to be close to 50% heads and 50% tails, as it will by chance. But how many times is "lots of times"? That is the question of sample size: How large does a study have to be to equalize confounding factors between groups reasonably well? Large enough to answer the question being asked, but this does not mean that all studies should be huge, or that larger is always better. At the very least, that attitude will have ethical problems, since many people may be unnecessarily exposed to research risks when a small number would have answered the question. With this background, as the saying goes, "A study needs to be as large as it needs to be." Not larger, and not smaller.

Put another way, we don't want a study to have unequal confounding factors in two groups despite randomizing patients to those two groups. This can happen by chance; just because we randomize, it does not follow that two groups will be equal in confounding factors. The more patients we randomize, however, the more likely that the two groups will be equal in confounding factors. The question is: How much more?

The Central Limit Theorem

There are two ways to answer this question: one clinical and one mathematical.

Clinically, to limit ourselves to psychiatric research, given moderate effect sizes for often subjective variables (like improvement in depressive symptom scores), one might generalize to say that at least 25 patients are needed per arm to detect a moderate effect size difference between groups. (Confounding factors could still impact the results, though.)

Mathematically, one might turn to the concept of the "central limit theorem." Stated mathematically, this means that "if you have an average, it should have a normal sampling distribution." In other words, the idea here is that if you obtain the average of a number of observations, then that average will be normally distributed after a certain number of observations. Getting back to our coin flip, two observations (flipping the coin just twice) is unlikely to give us a common average of 50% heads and 50% tails: the sample will not be normally distributed. On the other hand, 1,000 observations will be normally distributed, with the most common observation being 50% likely heads and 50% likely tails, and infrequent observations of extremes in either direction (mostly heads or mostly tails). So, the central limit theorem comes down to this: How many times do you have to flip a coin to get a normal distribution of observations (where the most common observation is 50% head and tails, and there are equal frequencies of observing either extreme?) The answer seems to be about n = 50.

Thus, whether clinically or mathematically, we come up with a figure of about 50 patients as being the cut-off for a large versus a small randomized study (hence the rationale for this figure in Table 3.1).

Interpreting Small RCTs

If the sample size is too small (<50), what are we to make of the RCT? In other words, if someone conducts a double-blind placebo-controlled RCT of 10 or 20 or 30 patients, what are we to make of it?

Basically, since it is highly likely that confounding factors will be unequal between groups, my view is that small RCTs should be seen as observational studies: they are perhaps slightly better in that they should not be *as* biased as a standard observational study, yet they *are* still biased. Hence, they cannot be taken at face value.

Even if a Table One showed that some measured variables are equal between groups in a small RCT, unmeasured confounders are still likely that could influence the results.

Also, because they are small, such RCTs cannot be adequately assessed through statistical analyses, like regression models, to reduce confounding bias (see Chapter 6). Their results simply have to stand on their own, as neither valid nor invalid, and as potentially meaningful but, equally, potentially meaningless.

Two Clinical Examples of Small RCTs

Here is an example of a small RCT that is possibly useful but, equally, possibly meaningless. Researchers wanted to show that serotonin reuptake inhibitor (SRI) antidepressants were effective in type II bipolar disorder (Parker et al. 2006). They gave citalopram by itself (without mood stabilizers) versus placebo to nine patients for three months; then, those who had received one arm of treatment were switched to the other treatment for three months; they were then switched back to the original treatment for another three months. The switching of treatments reflects a crossover design, but most relevant for our discussion is that the "randomization" initially involved four patients getting one treatment and five patients getting another. This obviously is nowhere near the number of repetitions that is required to equalize the two groups on most possible confounding factors. In the case of crossover studies, patients can, in a sense, serve as their own controls, as they are switched successively to drug versus placebo. So, this study had more rationale than if it had been a simple parallel-design study (e.g., four patients get drug versus five patients who get placebo, without any further changes). But, even with the crossover component, a study of this size is somewhat of a *glorified observational study*, and thus benefit with the drug would only be somewhat more impressive than in an observational report.

Another example is a study I conducted with my colleagues, assessing the efficacy of divalproex, an anticonvulsant, in acute bipolar depression (Ghaemi et al. 2007). The clinical lore is that this drug is ineffective in this setting. We gave it to 20 patients versus placebo, in a double-blind RCT, and we showed benefit. The study was not underpowered – that is, the small sample size did not lead to low statistical power, because our result was positive. Lack of statistical power is only relevant for negative studies (see next chapter). However, the positive result may have been biased by the small sample due to unsuccessful randomization, which is likely the case. Was the study worth doing?

The key is to avoid ivory-tower EBM (Chapter 16). One should not compare a study to the ideal design (all studies should then have one million patients and be triple-blind and placebo-controlled); one should compare a study to the best available evidence in the literature, asking the question "Does the study advance our current knowledge?" In this case, since there were only two prior small RCTs (one unpublished and negative, and one published and positive), our results at least pushed the literature a few inches in the positive direction.

One cannot infer definitive causation (see Chapter 14), but our study added (albeit in a limited way) to our knowledge and would lead us to continue to seek to see if this drug works in this condition with more studies (while a negative study might have led to less rationale for further research on this topic).

"Table One"

I mentioned that success of randomization needs to be assessed by a "Table One" which compares clinical and demographic variables in the two randomized groups. Some key concepts are needed to construct and interpret such a table. First, such tables should *never* have p-values. This is because, as described in the next chapter, RCTs are *not* designed to assess the relative frequency of males or females (or Republicans vs Democrats, or a host of other potential confounding factors) in the two groups; RCTs are designed to answer some question like whether a drug is more effective than placebo. That is the hypothesis the study is designed to test, not the frequency of 100 potential confounding variables. If p-values are used, their being positive is meaningless (due to false positive results given multiple comparisons; see Chapter 7), and their being negative is meaningless (due to false negative results since the sample may be too small, and the study was not designed to detect small differences between groups; see Chapter 7). Thus, no p-values should be used at all in Table One to distinguish potential confounding factors between two groups. Without p-values, how are we then supposed to tell if the two groups differ enough in a variable such that it might exert a *confounding* effect? If a study has 51% males and 49% females, is that enough of a difference to be a confounding effect? What if it is 52% males, 48% females? 53 vs 47%? 55 vs 45%? Where is the cut-off where we should be concerned that randomization might have failed, that chance variation between groups on a variable might have occurred despite randomization?

The Ten Percent Solution

Here is another part of statistics that is arbitrary: we say that a 10% difference between groups is the cut-off for a potential confounding effect. Thus, since 10% of 50 is 5%, we would be concerned about a gender difference that is something like 55% vs 45% (plus or minus 5% from the median). Suppose 25% of one group in our sample had a history of hospitalization for the illness being studied (and thus could be seen as more severely ill than those without past hospitalization); if the other group had a 31% rate of past hospitalization, the difference between the two groups is 6%, and we would be concerned about a difference between the groups of even 3% (10% of the absolute rate, which is 25% in one group and 31% in another group, or around 30% overall), and thus we definitely would be concerned about the observed 6% difference between the groups in past hospitalization (31% − 25% = 6%). It may turn out, if we mistakenly did a p-value, that the p-value would be 0.22 (not statistically significant), but we do not care. This study was not designed or powered to differentiate the two groups on past hospitalization; this hypothesis was not made before the study was conducted; and thus a p-value hypothesis test for this difference is wrong to do. We just care about the absolute difference between the groups in this variable: it is bigger than a 10% relative difference between the groups, and thus it is a potential confounding factor.

Then what do we do? We have a potential confounding factor; our study is over; we have the randomized results. How does this imbalance in our Table One influence our results?

There are at least two ways one can handle identified potential confounding bias after an RCT is finished. The most common approach is to simply report the randomized results as observed, state that there might be residual confounding bias as identified in Table One in relation to variable Y (gender, or past hospitalization), and thus imply that the results need to be taken with a grain of salt: they have some risk of invalidity. The other approach would be to conduct a regression model with the variable in question included so as to see if the observed randomized results change or not (see Appendix). In other words, one could treat the RCT as if it was an observational study, and analyze it accordingly (with regression models). If there is no or minimal change in the randomized result, one could then say that the observed imbalance was minor and had no appreciable confounding effect on the randomized study outcomes.

Not All RCTs Are Created Equal

The point of all this discussion is that, too often, researchers conduct a randomized study, and report the results, and that is it. They *assume* that randomization was successful (even though the study might be small, or even though there might in fact be observed imbalances in Table One). One should not assume the success of randomization; one should show it. *Not all RCTs are created equal.* Readers should be aware of this fact, and even though RCTs should be viewed as more likely valid than other studies, they are not automatically valid; the success of randomization should always be the first question that is asked and answered before one begins to consider an RCT as potentially valid.

Clinical Trials: Improving on Clinical Experience

Chapter

6

The basic rationale for clinical trials is to remove confounding bias and thereby to clarify what is true and what is false in clinical experience. Unfortunately, most clinicians and also most researchers in psychiatry do not understand the concepts underlying clinical trials, and they either ignore or misinterpret them. This chapter will try to explain clinical trials conceptually and clarify common misunderstandings.

Randomized clinical trials (RCTs) are the main basis for clinical research. Many statistical methods have been developed or refined in the context of RCTs. As discussed earlier, the first official RCT by A. Bradford Hill was conducted in 1948 for miliary tuberculosis. Hill used Ronald Fisher's p-value method for the first time in humans, as opposed to the original application by Fisher for agriculture. Unlike plant seeds, which can be influenced by seasons, the weather, and other limited confounding factors, human beings themselves can influence outcomes through psychological means. Hence, RCTs in humans are more complicated than in plants, and all the more necessary, given the many confounding factors involved in human experience.

Clinical practice is confounded; hence, RCTs are needed to show the truth. These many human factors lead to a high rate of confounding bias in real-world clinical practice. Clinical practice is confounded, such that you cannot believe your eyes. RCTs are like prescription eyeglasses, clarifying the blurriness of real-world clinical practice and giving sharp vision so that clinicians can see what is causing what. RCTs are needed to show the truth.

Two examples will be discussed here about how RCTs clarify clinical practice and provide better vision to the blurred experience of clinicians: antidepressant efficacy in so-called "major depressive disorder" (MDD) and in bipolar depression.

Regarding antidepressant efficacy in MDD, a classic meta-analysis provides important lessons about how RCTs can show the truth, but also how they can be used to mislead. In the first meta-analysis from about a decade ago (Kirsch et al. 2008), the authors mainly wanted to claim that antidepressants are not effective. They made this claim by showing that the overall absolute effect size of benefit was small. This view was expressed by analyzing the hundreds of RCTs conducted by pharmaceutical companies using the Cohen's d statistic, which is defined as showing no difference at all if the score is 0, having a moderate effect size with a score of 0.5, and have a large effect size with a score of near 1.0 or above. Cohen defined the 0.5 cut-off as a proxy for some clinically meaningful effect. The meta-analysis showed that antidepressants as a whole, when averaged together, had an overall Cohen's d score of about 0.3 (Figure 6.1). Since that score is below the postulated clinically meaningful effect limit of 0.5, it was concluded that antidepressants had no clinically meaningful benefit.

In further analysis, though, this overall average effect size of 0.3 reflected a range from basically 0.0 in mild depression to above 0.5 in severe depression (see Figure 6.3).

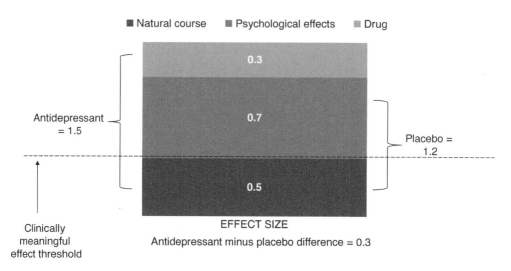

Figure 6.1 Absolute effect size for treatment of depression: 3 components

So, the more accurate description was that antidepressants had no efficacy at all in mild depression over placebo, but they had clinically meaningful benefit over placebo in severe depression. Hence, one simply cannot conclude that they "don't work," but rather that their effects vary based on severity.

Another interesting feature of that meta-analysis, as discussed later, is the distinction between absolute effect size and relative effect size. Figures 6.2 and 6.3 show exactly how valuable RCTs are over clinical experience. We observe that the reason why antidepressants are not better than placebo in mild depression, but notably better in severe depression, is not because antidepressants work better in severe depression, but rather because placebo is more effective in mild depression. This fact is well known, as discussed in Chapter 9. Placebo effect declines with severity. This phenomenon is well proven. This study merely replicates that reality, but the authors were interested in making judgments about antidepressants, not placebo. They concluded that antidepressants were less effective in mild depression, which is not true, rather than that placebo is more effective in mild depression, which is true.

In clinical experience, there is no placebo, so imagine the figure without the placebo line (Figure 6.2).

Recall that Cohen's d is defined as meaning that a large effect size of benefit is seen with scores nearing 1.0 or higher. The experience of the clinician is simply this line, which shows very large clinical benefit when antidepressants are given, and this benefit does not change whatever the severity of depression – mild, moderate, or marked. No wonder so many clinicians have been so enthusiastic about antidepressants. It's also the experience of patients. They feel better when they take the drugs.

Now look at the figure with the placebo arm alone (Figure 6.3).

This picture is something that is invisible to clinicians and patients. They do not know that what they are observing and experiencing is driven by this hidden reality. The placebo effect is large in mild illnesses, and it declines with severity. This scientific fact influences clinical experience. Notice that the placebo benefit for mild depression is huge, with Cohen's d around 1.0. Notice also that it is not the case that declining placebo benefit makes it useless

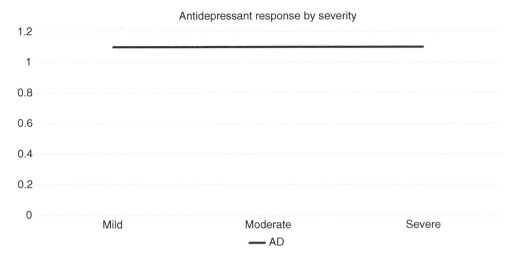

Figure 6.2 Clinical experience: Antidepressants work!

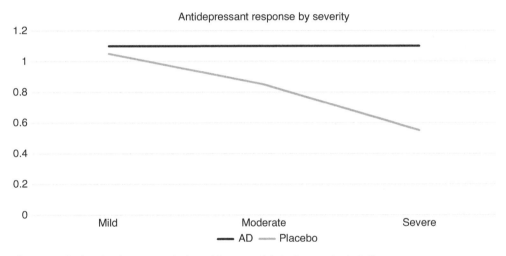

Figure 6.3 Reality: Antidepressants don't work because of their pharmacological effects

in severe depression. Even there, placebo alone provides clinically meaningful benefit with Cohen's d above 0.5. Placebo should not be underestimated, but it is not what people often think, as discussed in Chapter 9.

Now return to the original picture. Patients improve in mild depression markedly, but it's not because of the pharmacological effects of serotonin reuptake inhibition. It's because of placebo, which reflects something else. They still improve in moderate to severe depression, with clinically meaningful benefit from both placebo and the pharmacological effects of the antidepressants. To clinicians and patients, all they see and observe is consistent improvement in all cases with antidepressant. But RCTs clarify this blurred vision of clinical experience to show why patients improve: sometimes it's because of the medications, sometimes it's not.

Another example of the same phenomenon has to do with RCTs of antidepressant efficacy in bipolar depression. Again, there is a major disconnect between clinical practice and RCT evidence. Clinicians believe that antidepressants are effective in bipolar depression and, despite two decades of continual research showing their lack of efficacy, antidepressant treatment rates in bipolar depression have not declined. About half of all patients with bipolar illness are treated with antidepressants, and this rate has remained stable for the past two decades, even increasing somewhat in recent years. This class of medication ranks second in frequency of usage for this illness (behind antipsychotics) despite being completely ineffective. In contrast, the agents most proven to be effective – standard mood stabilizers such as lithium and divalproex – are the least used (given only to about one-third of patients). What explains this contrast between scientific reality and clinical practice? Again, the answer is confounding bias, which blurs the vision of clinicians and patients.

An example of an RCT which proves the falsehood of clinical experience in this case is the recent CAPE-BD study, conducted by our research group. In that study, patients were randomized to receive citalopram or placebo for an acute bipolar depressive episode, added to baseline treatment with standard mood stabilizers. The results of the main outcome are shown in Figure 6.4.

As can be seen, the antidepressant citalopram is clearly little different than placebo, with no clinically meaningful difference in benefit. As also can be seen, both curves show notable improvement, with more than 50% benefit in depression rating scores, which is the definition of clinical response. In other words, citalopram was ineffective for bipolar depression,

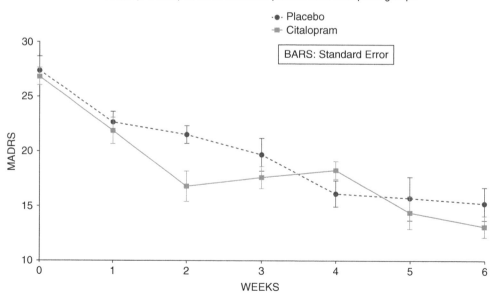

Figure 6.4 Antidepressant efficacy in bipolar depression: Clinicians see antidepressants work, but don't realize it's a placebo effect

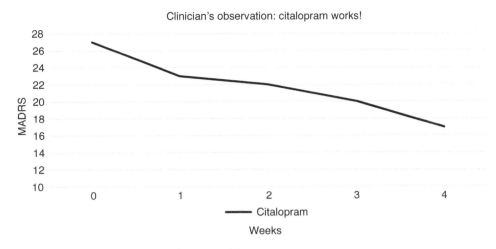

Figure 6.5 Clinician's observation: Citalopram works!

but not because it didn't make patients better. It made patients better; but it didn't make patients better than placebo. Put another way: citalopram worked, but not because of citalopram, not because of its pure serotonin reuptake inhibition. It worked because of the placebo benefits of any treatment.

Returning to the falsehood of clinical experience, one can imagine looking at that figure without the placebo arm and see why clinicians refuse to stop using antidepressants in bipolar depression (Figure 6.5).

Clinicians see improvement when they prescribe antidepressants in bipolar depression. Patients improve. The mistake made by clinicians is that they attribute that improvement to the treatment given – in this case, an antidepressant. They do not realize, as the full figure shows, that the improvement is entirely driven by placebo benefits unrelated to the pharmacological effects of the medication. RCTs reveal the truth. Clinical experience is blurred and misinterpreted. This is why clinical trials are so important in helping us better understand our clinical experience. It also is why clinicians need to change their practice once they are informed by RCTs. Yet they often don't, because they don't realize how RCTs can educate them about the confounding bias of their clinical experience.

The Use and Misuse of P-Values in Clinical Trials

Clinical trials generally are designed to answer a single question, but we humans force them to answer hundreds. This is the source of both their power and their debility.

The value of clinical trials comes from this ability to definitively (or as definitively as is impossible, in this inductive world) answer a single question: Does aspirin prevent heart attacks? Does streptomycin cure pneumonia? We want to know the answers. And each single answer, with nothing further said, is worth tons of gold to the health of humankind.

Such a single question is called the *primary outcome* of a clinical trial.

But we researchers and doctors and patients want to know more. Not only do we want to know if aspirin prevent heart attacks, we want to know if it also leads to lower death rates.

Did it prevent stroke too perhaps? What kinds of side effects did it cause? Did it cause gastrointestinal bleeding? If so, how many died from such bleeding?

So we seem forced to ask many questions of our clinical trials, partly because we want to know about side effects, but partly just out of our own curiosity: we want to know as much as possible about the effects of a drug on a range of possible benefits.

Sometimes we ask many questions for economic reasons. Clinical trials are expensive; whether a pharmaceutical company or the federal government is paying for it, in either case shareholders or taxpayers will want to get as much as possible out of their investment. You spent $10 million to answer one question? Could you not answer 5 more? Perhaps if you answered 50 questions, the investment would seem even more successful. This may be how it is in business, but in science the more questions you seek to answer, the fewer you answer well.

False Positives and False Negatives

The clinical trial is designed primarily to remove the problem of confounding bias – that is, to give us valid data. It removes the problem of bias, but is then faced with the problem of chance.

Chance can lead to false results in two directions: false positives and false negatives. False positives occur when the p-value is abused. If too many p-values are assessed, then the actual values will be incorrect. An inflation of chance error occurs, and one will be likely to observe many chance positive findings.

False negatives occur when the p-value is abnormally high due to excessive variability in the data. What this means is that there are not enough data points – not enough patients – to limit the variation in the results. The higher the variation, the higher the p-value. Thus, if a study is too small, it will be highly variable in its data – that is, it will lack precision and the p-value will be inflated. Therefore, the effect will be deemed statistically unworthy.

A false positive error is also called a *type I or alpha error*; a false negative is called a *type II or beta error*. The ability to avoid false negative results by having limited variability and higher precision of the data is called *statistical power*.

To avoid both of these kinds of errors, the clinical trial needs to establish a single, primary outcome. By essentially putting all its eggs in one basket, the trial is stating that the p-value for that single analysis should be taken at face value; it will not be distorted by multiple comparisons. Further, by having a primary outcome, the clinical trial can be designed such that a large enough sample size is calculated to limit the variability of the data, improve the precision of the study, and ensure a reasonable likelihood of statistical significance if a certain effect size is obtained.

A clinical trial rises and falls on careful selection of a primary outcome, and careful design of the study and sample size so as to assess the primary outcome.

The Primary Outcome

The primary outcome is usually some kind of measurement, such as points on a depression rating scale. This measurement can be defined in various ways; for example, it can reflect the actual change in points on a depression rating scale with drug versus placebo, or it can reflect the percentage of responders in drug versus placebo groups (usually defining response as 50% or more improvement in depression rating scale score). In general, the first approach is taken: the actual change in points is compared in the two groups. This is a continuous scale of measurement (1, 2, 3, 4 points . . .) not a categorical scale (responders versus nonresponders), which is a strength. Statistically, continuous measurements provide more data, less variability, and thus more statistical power, thereby enhancing the possibility of a lower p-value. This is the main reason why most primary outcomes in psychiatry and psychology involve continuous rating scale measures.

On the other hand, categorical assessments are often intuitively more understandable by clinicians. Thus, it is typical for a clinical treatment study in psychiatry to be designed mainly to describe a change in depressive symptoms as a number (a continuous change), while also to report the percentage of responders as a second outcome. While both of these outcomes flow one from the other, it is important for researchers to make choice; they cannot both equally be primary outcomes. A primary outcome is one outcome, and only one outcome. The other is a secondary outcome.

Secondary Outcomes

It is natural to want to answer more than one question in a clinical trial. But one needs to be clear which questions are secondary ones, and they need to be distinguished from the primary question. Their results, whether positive or negative, need to be equally interpreted more cautiously than in the case of the primary outcome.

Yet, it is not uncommon to see research studies where the primary outcome, such as a continuous change in a depression rating score, may not show a statistically significant benefit, while a secondary outcome, like categorical response rate, may do so. Researchers then may be tempted to emphasize the categorical response throughout the paper and abstract.

Not only can secondary outcomes be falsely positive, they can just as commonly be falsely negative. In fact, secondary analyses should be seen as inherently underpowered. An analysis found that, after the single primary outcome, the sample size needed to be about 20% larger for a single secondary outcome, and 30% larger for two secondary outcomes (Leon 2004).

Post-Hoc Analyses and Subgroup Effects

We now reach the vexed problem of subgroup effects. This is the place where, perhaps most directly, statisticians and clinicians have opposite goals. A statistician wants to get results that are as valid as possible and as far removed from chance as possible. This requires isolating one's research question more and more cleanly, such that all other factors can be controlled and the research question answered directly. A clinician wants to treat the individual patient in front of them, a patient who usually has multiple characteristics (each of us belongs to a certain race, has a certain gender, an age, a social class, a specific history of medical symptoms, and so on) and where the clinical matter in question occurs in the context of those multiple characteristics. The statistician produces an answer for the average patient on an isolated question; the clinician wants an answer for a specific patient with multiple relevant features that influence the clinical question. For the statistician, the question might be "Is antidepressant X better than placebo in the average patient?" For the clinician, the question might be "Is antidepressant X better than placebo in this specific patient who is African-American, male, 90 years old, with comorbid liver disease?" Or, alternatively, "Is antidepressant X better than placebo in this specific patient who is white, female, 20 years old, with comorbid substance abuse?" Neither of them is the "average" patient, if there is such a thing: one would have to imagine a middle-aged person with multiple racial complexity and partial comorbidities of varying kinds.

In other words, if the primary outcome of a clinical trial gives us the "average" result in an "average" patient, how can we apply those results to specific patients? The most common approach, for better and for worse, is to conduct subgroup analyses. In the example given earlier, we might look at the antidepressant response in men versus women, whites versus blacks, old versus young, and so on. Unfortunately, these analyses are usually conducted with p-values, which leads to both false positive and false negative risks, as noted earlier.

The Inflation of P-Values

To briefly reiterate, because this matter is worth repeating over and over: the false positive risk is that repeated analyses are a misapplication of the size of the p-value. A p-value of 0.05 means that with one analysis one has a 5% likelihood that the observed result occurred by chance. If 10 analyses are conducted, one of which produces a p-value of 0.05, that does NOT mean that the likelihood of that result by chance is 5%; rather, it is nearer to 40%. That is the whole concept of a p-value: If analyses are repeated enough, false positive chance findings will occur at a certain frequency, as shown in Table 6.1 for a computer simulation by my colleague Eric Smith (personal communication 2008).

Suppose we are willing to accept a p-value of 0.05, meaning that, assuming the null hypothesis is true, the observed difference is likely to occur by chance 5% of the time. The chance of inaccurately accepting a positive finding (rejecting the null hypothesis) would be 5% for one comparison, about 10% for 2 comparisons, 22% for 5 comparisons, and 40% for 10 comparisons. This means that if in an RCT the primary analysis is negative, but one of 4 secondary analyses is positive with p = 0.05, then that p-value actually reflects a 22% false positive chance finding, not a 5% false positive chance finding. And we would not accept

Table 6.1 Inflation of false positive probabilities with outcomes tested

Number of hypotheses tested	Type I error tested at 0.05 level
1	0.05
2	0.0975
3	0.14
5	0.23
10	0.40
15	0.54
20	0.64
30	0.785
50	0.92
75	0.979
100	0.999

that higher chance likelihood. Yet, clinicians and researchers often do not consider this issue. One option would be to do a correction for multiple comparisons, such as the Bonferroni correction, which would require that the p-value be maintained at 0.05 overall by dividing it by the number of comparisons made. For 5 comparisons, the acceptable p-value would be 0.05/5, or 0.01. The other approach would be to simply accept the finding, but to give less and less interpretive weight to a positive result as more and more analyses are performed.

This is the main rationale why, when a randomized clinical trial (RCT) is designed, researchers should choose one or a few primary outcome measures for which the study should be properly powered (a level of 0.80 or 0.90 [power = 1 – type II error] is a standard convention). Usually there is a main efficacy outcome measure, with one or two secondary efficacy or side-effect outcome measures. An efficacy effect or side effect to be tested can be established either a priori (before the study, which is always the case for primary and secondary outcomes) or post hoc (after the fact, which should be viewed as exploratory and not confirmatory of any hypothesis).

The Astrology of Subgroup Analysis

One cannot leave this topic without describing a classic study about the false positive risks of subgroup analysis, an analysis which correlated astrological signs with cardiovascular outcomes. In this famous report, the investigators for a well-known study of anti-arrhythmic drugs (ISIS-2) decided to do a subgroup analysis of outcome by astrological sign (Sleight 2000). (The title of the paper was: "Subgroup analyses in clinical trials: fun to look at – but don't believe them!") The trial was huge, involving about 17,000 patients, and thus some chance positive findings would be expected with enough analyses in such a large sample. The primary outcome of the study was a comparison of aspirin versus streptokinase for prevention of myocardial infarction, with a finding in favor of aspirin. In subgroup analyses by astrological sign, the authors found that patients born under Gemini or Libra experienced "a slightly adverse effect of aspirin on mortality (9% increase, SD 13; NS), while for patients born under all other astrological signs there was a striking beneficial effect (28% reduction, SD 5; $2p < 0.00001$)."

Either there is something to astrology, or subgroup analyses should be viewed cautiously.

It will not do to only think of positive subgroup results as inherently faulty, however. The false negative risk is just as important; p-values above 0.05 are often called "no difference," when in fact one group can be twice as frequent or larger than the other; yet if the overall frequency of the event is low (as it often is with side effects; see section on "Side Effects"), then the statistical power of the subgroup analyses will be limited and p-values will be above 0.05. Thinking of how sample size affects statistical power, note that with subgroup analyses samples are being chopped up into smaller groups, and thus statistical power declines notably.

So, subgroup analyses are both falsely positive and falsely negative, and yet clinicians will want to ask those questions. Some statisticians recommend holding the line, and refusing to do subgroup analyses. Unfortunately, patients are living people who demand the best answers we can give, even if they are not nearly certain beyond chance likelihood. Let us examine some of the ways statisticians have suggested that the risks of subgroup analyses can be mitigated.

Legitimizing Subgroup Analyses

Two common approaches follow:

1. Divide the p-value by the number of analyses; this will provide the new level of statistical significance. Called the "Bonferroni correction," the idea is that if 10 analyses are conducted, then the standard for significance for any single analysis would be 0.05/10 = 0.005. The higher threshold of 0.5%, rather than 5%, would be used to call a result unlikely to have happened by chance. This approach draws the p-value noose as tight as possible so that what passes through is likely true, but much that is true fails to pass through. Some more liberal alternatives (like the Tukey test) exist, but all such approaches are guesses about levels of significance, which can be either too conservative or too liberal.

2. Choose the subgroup analyses before the study, a priori, rather than post-hoc. The problem with post-hoc analyses is that, almost always, researchers do not report how many such analyses were conducted. Thus, if a report states that subgroup analysis X found a p = 0.04, we do not know if it was one of only 5, or one of 500, analyses conducted. As noted, there is a huge difference in how we would interpret that p-value depending on the denominator of how many times it was tested in different subgroup analyses. By stating a priori, before any data analysis occurs, that we plan to conduct a subgroup analysis, that suspicion is removed for readers. However, if one states that one plans to do 25 a priori subgroup analyses, those are still subject to the same inflation of p-value false positive findings as noted earlier.

In the *New England Journal of Medicine*, the most highly read medical journal, which is generally seen as having among the highest statistical standards, a review of 95 randomized clinical trials published therein found that 61% conducted subgroup analyses (Wang et al. 2007). Of these 51 RCTs with subgroup analyses, 43% were not clear about whether the analyses were a priori or post hoc, and 67% conducted 5 or more subgroup analyses. Thus, even in the strictest medical journals, about half of all subgroup analyses are not reported clearly or conducted conservatively.

Some authors also point out that subgroup analyses are weakened by the fact that they generally examine features that may influence results one by one. Thus, antidepressant response is compared by gender, then by race, then by social class, and so on. This is equivalent, as described previously, to univariate statistical comparisons as opposed to multivariate analyses. The problem is that women may not differ from men in antidepressant response, but perhaps white women differ from African-American men, or perhaps white older women differ from African-American younger men. In other words, multiple clinical features may go together and, as a group but not singly, influence the outcome. These possibilities are not captured in typical subgroup effect analyses. Some authors recommend, therefore, that after an RCT is complete, multivariate regression models be conducted in search of possible subgroup effects. Again, while clinically relevant, this approach still will have notable false positive and false negative risks.

In sum, clinical trials do well in answering the primary question which they are designed to answer. Further questions can only be answered with decreasing levels of confidence with standard hypothesis-testing statistics. As described later, I will advocate that these limitations make the use of hypothesis-testing statistics irrelevant, and that we should turn to descriptive statistical methods instead in looking at clinical subgroups in RCTs.

Power Analysis

Most authors focus on the false positive risks of subgroup analyses. But important false negative risks also exist. This brings us to the question of statistical power. We might define this term as the ability of the study to identify the result in question; to put it another way, how likely is the study to note that a difference between two groups is statistically significant? Power depends on three factors, two of which are sample size and variability of data. Most authors focus on sample size, but data variability is just as relevant. In fact, the two factors go together: the larger the sample, the smaller the data variability; the smaller the sample, the larger the data variability. The benefit of large samples is that, as more and more subjects are included in a study, the results become more and more consistent: everybody tends toward getting the same result; hence, there is less variability in the data. The typical measure of the variability of the data is the standard deviation (which is the standard error squared).

The third factor, also frequently ignored, is the effect size: the larger the effect size, the greater the statistical power of the study; the smaller the effect size, the lower the statistical power. Sometimes, an effect of a treatment might be so strong and so definitive, however, that even with a small sample the study subjects tend to consistently get the same result, and thus the data variability is also small. In that example, statistical power will be rather good even though the sample size is small, as long as there is a large effect size and a low standard deviation.

In contrast, a highly underpowered study will have a small effect size, high data variability (large standard variation), and a small sample size. We often face this latter circumstance in the scenario of medication side effects.

The equation used to calculate statistical power reflects the relationships between these three variables:

Statistical power (or beta; see section on "Power Analysis") = Effect size × sample size / standard deviation

Thus, the larger the numerator (large sample, large effect size) or the smaller the denominator (small standard deviation), the larger the statistical power.

The mathematical notation used for statistical power is "beta," with beta error reflecting the false negative risk (just as "alpha" error reflects the false positive risk – i.e., the p-value, as discussed previously). Beta reflects the probability of not rejecting the alternative hypothesis (the idea that the null hypothesis is false – i.e., a real difference exists in a study) when the alternative hypothesis is true. The contrast with the p-value or alpha error is that alpha is the probability of rejecting the null hypothesis when the null hypothesis is true.

As discussed previously, the somewhat arbitrary standard for false positive risk, or alpha error, is 5% (p or alpha = 0.05). We are willing to mistakenly reject the null hypothesis (NH) up to the point where the data are 95% or more certain to be free from chance occurrence. The equally arbitrary standard for beta error is 80% (Beta = 0.80): we are willing to mistakenly reject the alternative hypothesis (AH) up to the point where the data are 80% or more certain to be free from chance occurrence. Note that standard statistical practice is to be willing to risk false negatives 20% of the time, but false positives only 5% of the time: in other words, a higher threshold is placed on saying that a real difference exists in the data (rejecting the NH) than is placed on saying that no real difference exists in the data (rejecting the AH). This is another way of saying that statistical standards are biased toward more false negative findings than false positive findings. Why? There is no real reason.

One might speculate, in the case of medical statistics, that it matters more if we are wrong when we say that differences exist (e.g., that treatments work) than when we say that no differences exist (e.g., that treatments do not work), because treatments can cause harm (side effects) and thus we want to be rather certain that they work when we say they work.

The Subjectivity of Power Analysis

Although many statisticians have made a fuss about the need to conduct power analyses and how many research studies are not sufficiently powered to assess their outcomes, in practice power analysis can be a rather subjective affair – a kind of quantitative hand-waving. For instance, suppose I want to show that drug X will be better than placebo by a 25% difference in a depression rating scale. Using standard power calculations, I need to know two things to determine my needed sample size: the hypothesized difference between drug and placebo (the effect size), and the expected standard deviation (the variability of the data). For an acceptable power estimate of 80% (for Beta), and an expected effect size of 25% difference between drug and placebo, one gets quite differing results depending on how one estimates the standard deviation. Here, one needs to convert estimates to absolute numbers: Suppose the depression rating scale improvement was expected to be 10 points with drug; 25% difference would mean that placebo would lead to a 7.5 point improvement. The mean difference between the two groups would be 2.5 points (10 – 7.5). Standard deviation is commonly assessed as follows: If it is equal to the actual mean, then there is notable (but acceptable) variability; if it is smaller than the actual mean, then there is not much variability; if it is larger than the actual mean, then there is excessive variability. Thus, if we use a mean change of 7.5 points in the drug group as our standard, a good standard deviation would be about 5 (not much variability, most patients responded similarly), acceptable but bothersome would be 7.5, and too much variability would be a standard deviation of 10 or more. Using these different standard deviations in our power analysis produces rather different results (internet-based sample size calculators can easily be used for these calculations; I used www.stat.ubc.ca/~rollin/stats/ssize/n2.html [accessed August 22, 2008]): With low SD = 5, the above power analysis produces a needed sample size of 126; with medium SD = 7.5, the sample needed would be 284; and with high SD = 10, the sample needed would jump massively to 504. Which should we pick? As a researcher with limited resources or trying to convince an agency or company to fund my study, I would try to produce the lowest number, and I could do so by claiming a low standard deviation. Do I really know beforehand that the study will produce low variability in the data? No. It might; it might not. It may turn out that patients respond quite differently, and if the SD is large, then my study will turn out to be underpowered. One might deal with this problem by routinely picking a middle-range SD, like 7.5 in this example; but few researchers actually plan for the worst-case scenario, with a large SD, which would make many studies infeasibly large and in some cases overpowered (if the study turns out to have less variability than in the worst-case scenario).

The point of this example is to show that there are many assumptions that go into power analysis, based on guesswork, and that the process is not simply based on "facts" or hard data.

Side Effects

As a corollary of the need to limit the number of p-values, a common error in assessing the results of a clinical trial or observational study is to evaluate side effects across patient groups based on whether or not they differ on p-values (e.g., drug vs. placebo group). However, most clinical studies are not powered to assess side effects, especially when side effects are not frequent. Significance testing is not appropriate, since the risk of a false negative finding using this technique in isolation is too high.

Side effects should not be interpreted based on p-values and significance testing because of the high false negative (type II) error risk. They are not hypotheses to be tested, but simply observations to be reported. The appropriate statistical approach is to report the effect size (e.g., percent) with 95% confidence intervals (the range of expected estimated observations based on repeated studies).

These issues are directly relevant to the question of whether a drug has a risk of causing mania. In the case of lamotrigine, for instance, a review of the pooled clinical trials failed to find a difference with placebo, and reported no difference (Table 6.2).

Those studies were not designed to detect such a difference. It may indeed be that lamotrigine is not of higher risk than placebo, but it is concerning that the overall risk of pure manic episodes (1.3%) is four-fold higher than placebo (0.3%) (RR = 4.14, 95% CI 0.49–35.27): in fact, the sample size required to "statistically" detect (i.e., using "significance hypothesis testing" procedures) this observed difference in pure mania would be achieved with a study comparing two arms of almost 1,500 patients each (at a type II error level of 0.80, with statistical assumptions of no dropouts, perfect compliance, and equal-sized arms).

To give another example, if we accept a spontaneous baseline manic-switch rate of about 5% over two months of observation, and further assume that the minimal "clinically" relevant difference to be detected is a doubling of all events at a 10% rate in the lamotrigine group, the required sample size of a study properly powered to "statistically" detect this "clinically" significant difference should be almost 1,000 overall (assuming no dropouts, perfect compliance, and equal-sized arms). Only with such a sample could we be confident enough that a reported p-value greater than 0.05 really reflects a substantial, clinical

Table 6.2 Treatment-emergent mood events: All controlled studies to date

	Lamotrigine[*] (n = 314)	Placebo[**] (n = 314)	Test Statistic	Relative Risk	95% Confidence Intervals
Hypomania	2.1%	1.9%	$x^2 = 0.01, p = 0.93$	1.10	0.39–3.15
Mania	1.3%	0.3%	$x^2 = 1.01, p = 0.32$	4.14	0.49–35.27
Mixed episode	0.3%	0.3%	$x^2 = 0.33, p = 0.56$	0.83	0.05–13.19
All events	3.7%	2.5%	$x^2 = 0.41, p = 0.52$	1.45	0.62–3.41

* Bipolar disorder, n = 232, unipolar disorder, n = 147.
** Bipolar disorder, n = 166, unipolar disorder, n = 148.
From Ghaemi et al. (2003) with permission.

equivalence of lamotrigine and placebo in causing acute mania. These pooled data involved 693 patients, which is somewhat more than half the needed sample, but even larger samples would be needed due to the statistical assumptions requiring no dropouts, full compliance, and equal sample size in both arms.

The methodological point is that one cannot assume no difference when studies are not designed to test a hypothesis.

The Problem of Dropouts and Intent-to-Treat Analysis

Even if patients agree to participate in RCTs, one cannot expect that they will remain in those studies until the end. Humans are humans: they may change their minds, they might move away, or they might just get tired of coming to appointments; they could also have side effects or stop treatment because they are not getting better. Whatever the cause, when patients cannot complete an RCT, major problems arise in interpreting the results. The solution to the problem is usually the use of intent-to-treat (ITT) analyses.

What this means is that randomization equalizes all potential confounding factors for the entire sample at the beginning of the study. If that entire sample is analyzed at the end of the study, there should be no confounding bias. However, if some of that sample is not analyzed at the end of the study (as in a more complete analysis, where dropouts before the end of the study are not analyzed), then one cannot be sure that the two groups at the end of the study are still equal on all potential confounding factors. If some patients drop out of one treatment arm because of less efficacy, or more side effects, then these nonrandom dropouts will bias the ultimate results of the study in a more complete analysis. Thus, in general, an ITT approach is what is used. From the study design perspective, this is called ITT because we intend to treat all the patients for the entire duration of the study, whether or not they stay in the study until the very end. From the statistical analysis perspective, this is called the last-observation-carried-forward (LOCF) approach because it comes down to taking the last data point available for the patient and pretending that it occurred at the very end of the study. The problem with this approach is that it obviously assumes that the last outcome for the patient in the study would have remained the same until the very end of the study – that is, that the patient would not have gotten any better or any worse. This is less of a problem in a short-term as opposed to a maintenance study. Nonetheless, it is important to realize that there are assumptions built into both LOCF and more complete analyses and that none of them fully remove all possibility of bias.

Intent-to-treat analysis, like so much of statistics, is not perfect, but it is the best approach we have: it minimizes bias more than other approaches. It is a means to deal with the fact that humans are not animals, and that RCTs cannot possibly lead to absolute environmental control. We may randomize patients to a treatment but, unless we wish to go Stalinist, we cannot force them to remain on that treatment. The statistician who developed it, Richard Peto, realized its limitations while also realizing its value. As summarized by Salsburg:

> This approach may seem foolish at first glance. One can produce scenarios in which a standard treatment is being compared to an experimental one, with patients switched to the standard if they fail. Then, if the experimental treatment is worthless, all or most of the patients randomized to it will be switched to the standard, and the analysis will find the two treatments the same. As Richard Peto made it clear in his proposal, this method of analyzing

the results of a study cannot be used to find that treatments are equivalent. It can only be used if the analysis finds that they *differ* in effect.   (Salsburg 2001a, p. 277)

In other words, the residual bias with ITT analysis should work against benefit with an experimental drug, and thus any benefit seen in an ITT analysis is not likely to have been inflated.

The presence of some potential for bias in even the best-crafted RCT means that one can never be completely certain that the results of any RCT are valid. This raises the need for replication with multiple RCTs to get closer to establishing causation.

Generalizability

A cost to the aforementioned efforts to conduct clinical trials efficiently is that one can enhance the study validity at the expense of generalizability: some use the terms "internal" versus "external" validity to make the same point.

After crossing the hurdles of confounding bias and chance, a reader might conclude that the results of a study are valid. The final step is to assess the scope of these valid results. We then move to the topic of generalizability, which is quite different from validity. For generalizability (sometimes called external validity, as opposed to internal validity), one should ask the following question: Given that these results are right, to whom do they apply? In other words, who was in the sample? More directly, clinicians might want to compare their own patients to those in the sample to determine which of their patients might be affected by what they learned from that study. To some extent, validity is a relative concept: for example, investigators observe that one group of patients does better than another. But generalizability is an absolute concept: How many patients did better? And who were those patients? One has to search the methods section carefully to answer this question, usually by looking for the "inclusion and exclusion criteria" of a study.

One way in which generalizability is discussed is often by using the term *efficacy* for the results of the samples of patients in clinical trials, and *effectiveness* for the results in larger populations of patients in the real world. "Services research" has developed as a field partly to emphasize the need for generalizable data obtained from nonclinical trial populations.

If patients have to go through all the hoops of randomization, blinding, placebo, rating scales, and so on, one might expect that only some patients would agree to participate in research studies with all those limitations. One study found that the simple use of placebo automatically excludes many patients: About half of patients with schizophrenia stated that they would refuse to participate in any study if it used placebo (Roberts et al. 2002; Hummer et al. 2003). Once one adds other demands of research (acceptance of randomization, frequent visits, blinding), one can expect that the majority of patients with major mental illnesses would refuse to participate in most RCTs. Then, when one adds the fact that there are always exclusion criteria, sometimes stringent, for all studies (often, for instance, exclusion of those with active substance abuse, or those who are noncompliant with appointments), then one may get the sense of how the RCT literature, which provides the most valid data and is the basis for most treatment decisions, is drawn from a small sliver of patients from the larger pie of persons with illnesses. One study of elderly depression found that only 4.2% of 188 severely depressed elderly patients were able to enter an antidepressant study (mostly due to exclusion due to concomitant psychiatric or medical illnesses) (Yastrubetskaya, Chiu, and O'Connell 1997). Another research group applied standard exclusion criteria in many antidepressant clinical trials (mainly psychiatric and substance abuse comorbidities or current suicidal ideation) to 293 patients whom they had diagnosed with a unipolar current major depressive episode in regular clinical practice (Zimmerman, Mattia, and Posternak 2002). They found that only 14% of patients would have met standard inclusion criteria for antidepressant clinical trials. Assuming that about one-half or so would simply refuse to take placebo or receive blinded treatment, one can estimate that less than 10% would ultimately have participated in antidepressant RCTs.

Perhaps that number is a valid estimate: for any major psychiatric condition, about 10% of patients with the relevant diagnosis will quality for and agree to participate in available RCTs. The assumption in the world of clinical trials is that the research conducted on this 10% is generalizable to the other 90%. This may or may not be the case, and there is no clear way to prove or disprove the matter. It is just another place where statistics has its limits, and where clinicians should use statistical data with judgment (rather than simply rejecting nor unthinkingly accepting them).

Clinical examples: Maintenance studies of bipolar disorder

An example of the issue of generalizability involves studies of combination therapy, often with an antipsychotic plus a standard mood stabilizer, versus mood stabilizer monotherapy in treatment of acute mania. Those studies tend to routinely show benefit with combination treatment, yet it is important to note that the majority of patients in those studies initially must fail to respond to mood stabilizer monotherapy. Thus, the comparison is between an already failed treatment (mood stabilizer monotherapy) and a new treatment (combination treatment). In one study of risperidone in mania (Sachs et al. 2002), about one-third of the sample had not been previously treated with mood stabilizer, and thus were not selected for mood stabilizer nonresponse. Those patients entered the study initially without any treatment. They were then randomized to mood stabilizer alone (lithium, valproate, or carbamazepine, based on patient/doctor preference) versus mood stabilizer plus risperidone. Much less benefit with risperidone was seen when patients were *not* preselected for having already failed mood stabilizer monotherapy. In sum, studies which tend to support combination therapy with antipsychotic plus mood stabilizer are likely only generalizable to those who have failed mood stabilizer monotherapy. One *cannot* conclude, as is often heard, that combination therapy with these two classes of drugs generally is more effective than mood stabilizers alone.

Here is another place where numbers do not stand alone, another example of where we need to use concepts in statistics rather than simply calculations. Sampling from the larger population is unavoidable; thus, one must accept the results of samples while also paying attention to any unique features that may make them less generalizable. A balance is required.

Summary

RCTs have revolutionized medicine, yet they have many limitations. This is a reason not to view them as sufficient unto themselves, as in ivory-tower evidence-based medicine, but it is not a reason to devalue them as unnecessary. The most important tool is knowledge so that RCTs can be adequately evaluated.

P-Values: Uses and Misuses

Should we just stop using p-values?

Some might think that a statistics book that makes this claim would have nothing more to say. But, in fact, it should be clear by now that there is much more to statistics than p-values (or hypothesis testing methods). In fact, statistics has little to do with p-values – or, more correctly, p-values have as much to do with statistics as alcohol has to do with sociability: too much of the former ruins the latter.

Background

The concept of the p-value comes from Ronald Fisher's work on randomization of crops for agriculture. p-Values are, in effect, a statistical attempt to solve the philosophical problem called *the problem of induction* (see Chapter 14). If we observe something, we can never be 100% certain that what we have observed actually happened. It is possible that other things influenced what we observed (confounding bias; this is perhaps the most important source of error in induction), and it is possible that we observed something that occurred by chance. As discussed further in Chapter 14, the philosopher David Hume had long identified this probabilistic nature of induction. We have seen that each day the sun rises, he said. Day after day, the sun rises. Yet we never have complete (absolute, 100%) certainty that the sun will rise tomorrow. It is highly, highly likely (one might say 99.99% probable) that the sun will rise tomorrow, and thus we can proceed with the inductive inference that the sun will rise tomorrow. However, this strong inference does not imply that we are absolutely certain that this will happen.

For practical purposes, the difference between 99.99% and 100% is unimportant. (For philosophical purposes it may matter, and much has been made of Hume's argument that one cannot infer absolute causation from induction.) Probably, 99.98% is also close enough to 100% that it should not matter that there is a 0.02% risk that the event observed might have occurred by chance. What about 99.97%? 99.96%? 99.0%? 98% 97,96, 95%? Aha! We have reached the magic number. Or, at least, this is the number that is generally viewed as magic in contemporary research: the p-value of 0.05, which reflects a 95% likelihood that an observed inductive inference did not occur by chance.

Perhaps the reader can appreciate that the cut-off point of 95% vs 96% or 94% or 99% is rather arbitrary. Fisher never states anywhere why he thinks the p-value of 0.05 is preferable to 0.06 or 0.04 or 0.01. Presumably, the number 5 is more pleasing to the eye than 4 or 6.

David Salsburg, a statistician who searched Fisher's articles and books for an origin to this concept, reports that he only finds one place (interestingly, for mental health professionals, it occurred in the 1929 *Proceedings of the Society for Psychical Research*) where Fisher ascribes to the p = 0.05 criterion, and there Fisher is clear that the decision is arbitrary:

> In the investigation of living beings by biological methods, statistical tests of significance are essential. Their function is to prevent us being deceived by accidental occurrences, due not to the causes we wish to study, or are trying to detect, but to a combination of many other circumstances which we cannot control. An observation is judged significant, if it would rarely have been produced, in the absence of a real cause of the kind we are seeking. It is a common practice to judge a result significant, if it is of such a magnitude that it would have been produced by chance not more frequently than once in twenty trials. This is an *arbitrary, but convenient*, level of significance for the practical investigator, but it does not mean that he allows himself to be deceived once in every twenty experiments. The test of significance only tells him what to ignore, namely all experiments in which significant results are not obtained.
> (Salsburg 2001a, p. 99 [italics added])

There is no scientific reason for p = 0.05 as opposed to others near it, and here the reader can note that an essential part of the edifice of statistics – this highly mathematical and scientific discipline – has absolutely no basis in science or mathematics at all. Statistics, like all human endeavors, is based, in part, on conceptual assumptions. It is not a science of positive facts through and through.

It is worth pointing out that earlier statisticians in the nineteenth century, though without using the actual phrase "p-value," had developed the concept that the influence of chance needed to be small in making statistical comparisons. How small? Bernoulli used the term "moral certainty" to apply to a likelihood of 1:1,000 or less ($p < 0.001$). Edgeworth suggested a level of certainty equivalent to a p-value of 0.005 (Stigler 1986, p. 311). Thus, one sees that earlier statisticians suggested a much stricter standard than has become current.

If we appreciate how this 0.05 criterion came about, we might also be more generous and less focused on whether a study result has a p-value of 0.05 or 0.055 (which, God forbid, rounds up to 0.06). I have seen researchers sweat and squirm as a data analysis produces a p-value of 0.06 – the study seems hardly publishable, and certainly less impactful, with that difference of 0.01 from the golden threshold of 0.05.

This is one reason to give less credence to p-values: the cut-off point is arbitrary. But arbitrariness does not imply incoherence. Obviously, a p-value above 0.50 (50% chance likelihood) would suggest a truly chance observation. In the lower range of p-values, small differences are not conceptually meaningful. For that reason, we should not treat p-values with reverence – as "mathematical substitutes for sensible thought" – seeking to obtain a magic number almost as if it were a talisman against error; rather, we should interpret p-values for what they are, use them when it makes sense, and refuse to abuse them.

With that context, we should now define what the p-value means. The p stands for probability, and the p-value may be defined as follow: *The probability of observing the observed data, assuming that the null hypothesis is true.* The p-value is not a real number; it does not reflect a real probability, but rather the likelihood of chance effects *assuming* (but not knowing) that the null condition is true: "It is a theoretical probability associated with observations under conditions that are most likely false. It has nothing to do with reality. It is an indirect measurement of plausibility" (Salsburg 2001a, p. 111). It is not the probability of an event, but the probability of our *certainty* about an event. Indeed, in this sense, it is a central expression of LaPlace's concept of statistics as quantifying, rather than disclaiming, our ignorance (Menand 2001). A p-value attempts to quantify our ignorance, rather than establish any reality.

Thus, if we use a standard p-value cut-off of 0.05 or less as the definition of *statistical significance*, what we are saying is that *we will be rejecting the null hypothesis by mistake 5% of the time or less.*

Note some important misunderstandings:

1. The p-value is *not* the probability of the null hypothesis being true.
2. The p-value is *not* the probability of the results occurring *by chance*; it is the probability of the observed results *really* being the case, *if* we assume the null hypothesis to be true.

The key relevance for the p-value, as originally developed by Fisher, is not the specific number, but the concept of rareness, the idea that one should examine how likely the play of chance could be, and to interpret one's results more definitively as the likelihood of chance becomes more and more rare. Salsburg notes:

> Reading through Fisher's applied papers, one is led to believe that he used significance tests to come to one of three possible conclusions. If the p-value is very small (usually less than .01), he declares that an effect has been shown. If the p-value is large (usually greater than .20), he declares that, if there is an effect, it is so small that no experiment of this size will be able to detect it. If the p-value lies in between, he discusses how the next experiment should be designed to get a better idea of the effect. (Salsburg 2001a, p. 100)

How p-Values Led to Hypothesis-Testing

Originally, in the 1920s, Fisher developed the p-value concept solely in relation to this notion of statistical significance. Within two decades, however, the use of the p-value and the concept of statistical significance were quickly tied to the concept of rejecting a null hypothesis. This evolution occurred through the joint efforts of Fisher's younger colleague Egon Pearson (the son of Fisher's nemesis, Karl Pearson) and the collaboration of Jerzy Neyman; hence, the hypothesis-testing approach, now standard in mainstream statistics, was originally called the Neyman-Pearson approach.

What Neyman and Pearson faced was the problem that Fisher's p-value seemed to sit in a conceptual void. We knew what it meant if it was very small: the observed results were unlikely to have occurred by chance. But what if a result was nonsignificant? Does this mean that "a hypothesis is true if we fail to refute it?" (Salsburg 2001a, p. 107). Recall that Fisher's view was that large p-values would suggest that one could not decide. He clearly stated that a nonsignificant result does not mean that any hypothesis was thereby proven: we might reject that there *is* a difference, but we have not thereby proven that there is *no* difference. Neyman and Pearson wanted to establish this idea more clearly. They concluded that significance testing with p-values needed to occur in a conceptual structure wherein two separate alternatives are present: the null hypothesis of no difference, and the alternative hypothesis of a difference. They introduced these now commonplace terms and, more importantly, the conceptual assumptions upon which our current mega-structure of medical statistics rests. They then defined the probability of detecting the alternative hypothesis as the "power" of a significance test. Now, p-values would not only need to reflect the probability for testing the null hypothesis, they also needed to provide a probability for testing the alternative hypothesis. The concept of power became central to defining a significance test, and false negatives, not just false positives, were better defined (Salsburg 2001a).

Fisher's development of p-values to quantify the probability of chance error in observations led to conceptual problems that Neyman and Pearson tried to solve by devising the concepts of null hypotheses, alternative hypotheses, and power. Fisher was not happy with the additional Neyman-Pearson approach to using p-values, but it has become consecrated now. Called hypothesis-testing, this approach is as central to modern statistics as the supply-and-demand concept is to modern economics. But, just as supply-and-demand economics is at best partially correct, and simply wrong in many ways, so too hypothesis-testing is only sometimes helpful in statistics, and often nothing but a source of confusion and error. Fisher's apprehensions have, frankly, proven true. (It may be relevant that Neyman, who lived into the 1970s, himself rarely used hypothesis-testing methods in his own work; he used confidence intervals, a concept he also originated, much more, as I will also advocate in Chapter 10.)

The relevance of these debates is that we need to realize that our statistical concepts are not themselves scientific facts, nor did they arrive to us from Mount Sinai. They are the result of debates which are not yet finished. We need to realize that the foregoing storyline is what happened that led to the first line of most elementary statistics textbooks today. If we don't understand how we got to where we are today, we will misunderstand that first line, and hence everything that follows.

Definition: What Is the Null Hypothesis?

Since today the definition of the p-value relies on the definition of the null hypothesis, let us define the latter.

The null hypothesis is an assumption about the nature of the world, required for the use of p-values. The assumption is that things in the world are the same, that they do not differ from each other, and that inductive inferences about relations between things in the world are wrong. Thus stated, we see another assumption at the core of the world of statistics.

In essence, statistics is based on a thought experiment: Let us imagine that nothing of interest was happening in the world. Every time we thought we saw something, every time that we thought some event in the world happened, and every time we thought one thing caused another thing, we would be wrong. The world is unchanging and conservative, always tending toward the negative: things are not happening, observed differences are not real, inferred relationships are wrong. This is the world of the null hypothesis (NH). Why should we make this assumption? Why not the opposite assumption? I have not found in the statistical literature a clear conceptual explanation about why the NH is preferable to the opposite thought experiment (the idea, perhaps, that we should accept all differences and relations and inferences that appear to us through induction as real, sometimes called the Alternative Hypothesis or AH). When comparing the two alternatives, one sees that one is conservative (the NH) and one is liberal (the AH). Why be conservative in science? One argument might be that conservatism is justified in science because we are wrong so often; the history of science might be invoked to show how repeatedly we have been mistaken in our scientific claims. Now that a mathematical method – statistics – has been developed to test scientific theories, it might be rational to use that method to get rid of all the dead wood, all the wrongness, of scientific speculation, as opposed to using statistics to more easily confirm all these ideas and observations that people claim. Another way of putting it, specifically relevant to medical statistics, might be this: Since statistics are influential, once statistics confirm a claim, then doctors and patients are going to be likely to change their practice: they may start using a drug, they may stop using it, they may change their diets, they may start treating children in a certain way, and so on. With these important practical consequences, one might claim that statistics should err on the side of caution, only approving claims when they are highly likely to be true.

This would be a good rationale for the NH, except for the fact that I simply made it up. Not that my invention of it at this time reduces its validity, but it is noteworthy that statisticians themselves have not gone to great lengths to justify the NH as the basis for hypothesis-testing statistics.

The classic description of the NH was given by Fisher, who wrote: "The null hypothesis is never proved or established, but is possibly disproved, in the course of experimentation. Every experiment may be said to exist only in order to give the facts a chance of disproving the null hypothesis" (Fisher 1947, p. 16). Thus, Fisher admits the essentially speculative character of the NH assumption, and he highlights its central role in the our conception of research.

The asymmetry of our concept of the NH is central: we can never prove it; we can perhaps disprove it. This problem leads to the need for *noninferiority* designs as the closest we can get to testing the null hypothesis. We are left with the uncomfortable fact that we cannot empirically (or statistically) test a key concept on which much of statistics rests.

The Conservatism Assumption

One should be conservative about how to interpret research studies, providing a similar rationale for putting the p-value cut-off at 95% as opposed to 90% or 80%.

Yet there is a cost to this conservatism. Suppose a life-saving treatment arises, but is studied in a sample too small to reach the p-value of 0.05, and instead the treatment leads to a p-value of 0.11. Further, let us suppose that we are God (or gods). We know that this drug is, in fact, quite effective; let us stipulate that it is much more effective than any other available treatment. Let us also stipulate that it treats a serious illness, and for each year it is not used let us state, being God, that we know that 1 million persons will die. Now, the statistician, not being God, would only assess the situation this way: First, we assume that the null hypothesis is true: that the treatment is ineffective. (Even though God would know this is not true in this case, we mortals always must assume it to be true.) There is an 11% likelihood that the observed treatment effect would have occurred by chance, and thus we have an 11% likelihood that we would incorrectly reject the null hypothesis. This 11% possibility of being wrong is too high for us to accept, thus we will continue believing in the NH – namely, that the treatment is ineffective.

To put it starkly, how many lives are worth a 6% increased risk (11% – 5%) of being wrong by chance? Now, this is obviously an extreme situation, and the assumption that we could know the absolute truth like God is obviously false; but the point of thought experiments such as this one, commonly used in academic philosophy, is to bring out our own assumptions, our own intuitions, and their limitations. The problem with the NH approach is that it will automatically be biased (if we wish to use that term, one could also say "weighted") against real findings, real differences, and effective treatments. In cases where such real observations make a major difference in the world, the NH might be too conservative.

One can make this point another way with another thought experiment: Suppose that we are not God, we are mortals, but we know nothing about p-values. We had never heard of them, and we had no awareness of the tradition of a 95% cut-off for chance findings to reject the NH. But we knew all about that terrible illness and its limited available treatments. If I were to tell you, under these circumstances, that this new treatment was extremely effective and that the evidence for this efficacy was 89% *not* likely to be due to chance, would you be inclined to begin using it?

Assumption After Assumption

So, our first assumption was that p-values should demonstrate that a result was likely to occur outside of chance at the 0.05 level. Our second assumption was that we should accept the null hypothesis and lean toward rejecting observed inferences unless that level of probability of chance findings is shown. These are the two major assumptions of hypothesis-testing methods in statistics. They have some merit, but they also have some weaknesses and, perhaps most importantly, they are not themselves based on scientific evidence (or any other stronger form of evidence, such as divine revelation). They are not assumptions that can be, or should be, enforced on humankind as simply right or wrong; rather, they are assumptions, nothing more or nothing less, and if we find them coherent and useful we can accept them, and if not we can reject them. Statistics, like any discipline of human knowledge, needs to think about its concepts instead of rejecting any attempts to question them.

Statistical Significance

Now we can examine this term – statistical significance – so widely used in medical research. It basically reflects the p-value cut-off at which the NH can be rejected. Unfortunately, the word "significance" has other uses in the English language outside of statistics, hence this short-hand for a statistical result of research is often manipulated for the sometimes less wholesome goals of the human beings who do the research.

Salsburg notes that the original use of the word statistically "significant" by Fisher differs from what it has become: "The word was used in the late-nineteenth-century English meaning, which is simply that the computation *showed or signified something*. As the English language entered the twentieth century, the word *significant* began to take on other meanings, until it developed its current meaning, implying *something very important*" (Salsburg 2001a, p. 98 [italics added]). I would emphasize that we need to remember the originally meaning of the term: to say that something is statistically significant is to say that *something happened*: the drug is doing something. It does not mean that *something important happened*: that the drug is doing something robustly. (The latter connotation of significance requires the use of the effect size concept; see Chapter 8.)

Perhaps the main problem with the concept of statistical significance, however, is that it gives one meaning ("not statistically significant") to a wide range of possible results (p-values ranging from 0.05 to 1.0). Thus, if we only focus on whether a study is statistically significant (SS) or not, then we will say that treatment X with a p-value of 0.07 is not SS and treatment Y with a p-value of 0.94 is also not SS. Yet in one case, the likelihood of a nonchance finding is 93% and in the other case it is 6%. Sometimes researchers use another English word – "trend" – to denote those findings that are close to 0.05 but just not quite there (often it is used for p-values between 0.05 and 0.10). Yet when a "statistical trend" is identified, researchers usually are apologetic about it, often feeling the need to explicitly state, in case the reader did not know the statistical meaning of the word "trend," that it is not SS (e.g., "a nonsignificant trend," or "a statistical trend that is not statistically significant"). I would not be too bothered by the use of the concept of a statistical trend if researchers were able to use the term nonapologetically, but the constant reference to being non-SS undercuts the value of pointing out a statistical trend. The other problem is that this approach only pushes back the problem of the arbitrary cut-off. A p-value of 0.11 is not even a trend, so it is completely meaningless.

In my view, p-values are bad enough; translating p-values into English words with vague meaning ("significance," "trend") is worse. The term "statistical significance" mostly causes confusion.

Another major problem with the term is that it has purely statistical meaning in relation to p-values. It has no meaning in any other way. Yet since the word "significance" in English means, roughly, something that is important, and thus the words "statistical significance" tend to be interpreted by doctors and clinicians as meaning, if present, that the results are important, and, if absent, that the results are not important. Yet, as will be see in Chapter 8, due to the inherent limitations of p-values, the results of a study may be false positive (and thus the apparently important SS results are in fact not important) or it may be false negative (and thus the apparently unimportant SS results are in fact important). Sometimes clinicians try to finesse this problem by talking about "clinical significance" as complementary to SS, using the term "clinical significance" as a synonym for the more precise term "effect size," which we discuss in Chapter 8. Yet this is uncommonly done, and the continuing multiplication of varieties of "significance" is only bound to lead to more confusion; one is reminded of the interminable quarrels of leftist parties and their varying definitions of the word "revolution." Perhaps George Orwell had it right: the English language is much more easily abused than used, and we should stick to simple and clear, not vague and abstract, uses of words.

The Scope of p-Values

There is another feature of p-values that deserves commentary. According to their originator, Ronald Fisher, p-values *should only be used for randomized clinical trials* (RCTs), not for any other kind of scientific research, and especially not for observational clinical studies in medicine (Salsburg 2001a, pp. 302–3). This view may seem odd; if true, it would invalidate most medical research. But I think Fisher was right, if he is properly understood. The reader will recall the Three Cs: the first is confounding bias, the *second* is chance (and the third is causation). p-Values assess chance; they should not be used unless bias is first removed. RCTs remove bias and thus allow us to skip the first C and move to assessing chance. This was Fisher's insight. Let's give the use of p-values outside of RCTs a name: *Fisher's fallacy.* And this is still where Fisher was correct: if we use p-values willy-nilly, on observational data, without making any effort to reduce confounding or other biases statistically (as with regression models), we are misusing p-values. We cannot assess the minute influence of chance when our data could be massively biased. This was in fact the scientific basis for Fisher's critique of the epidemiological evidence that linked cigarette smoking to lung cancer. If the options are as Fisher had them – either use p-values only in

RCTs, or use p-values without further qualification for any kind of study – then Fisher is correct. Where Fisher erred was in not realizing the utility of epidemiological methods to reduce bias in non-RCT settings; regression modeling came later, so Fisher could not have known about it, but these statistical methods allow us to reduce, though not remove, bias and thus go a long way toward passing the first step of the three Cs and then allowing us to use p-values to assess chance. This was Bradford Hill's argument in the cigarette smoking and cancer controversy (see Chapter 14), which laid the foundation of so much of the current medical research. One simply cannot do RCTs for every medical matter, and thus epidemiological methods are better than nothing, and provide us with more useful knowledge than simply guessing. This is the basic insight behind evidence-based medicine (EBM; see Chapter 16). Fisher could not foresee where this would go, and he did not appreciate the early signs of this approach to valid knowledge outside of RCTs. However, his warning is still an important one: Bias comes first, and if it is not removed in some sense (either by RCTs or statistical analyses like regression), then the application of p-values is meaningless. And, indeed, most of the psychiatric literature still suffers from Fisher's fallacy, and thus misuses p-values.

The Faulty Logic of Hypothesis-Testing

There is another important problem with the whole hypothesis-testing approach: it rests on faulty logic. I will briefly make this point here, and then discuss it in more detail later. The prominent statistician Jacob Cohen called it the "illusion of attaining improbability," which is "the widespread belief that the level of significance at which [the null hypothesis] is rejected, say.05, is the probability that it is correct or, at the very least, that it is of low probability" (Cohen 1994, p. 998). This logic can be described as follows:

"If the null hypothesis is correct, then these data are highly unlikely.
These data have occurred.
Therefore, the null hypothesis is highly unlikely."   *(Cohen 1994, p. 998)*

Cohen showed that this logic does not work because it involves probability, which becomes clear once we fill in the abstract data with concrete things:

"If a person is an American then he is probably not a member of Congress.
  (TRUE, RIGHT?)
This person is a member of Congress.
Therefore, he is probably not an American."   *(Cohen 1994, p. 998)*

As a senior figure in statistics, and one who put most of his effort into research in psychology, Cohen's reservations toward the end of his life have not been sufficiently appreciated:

We, as teachers, consultants, authors, and otherwise perpetrators of quantitative methods, are responsible for the ritualization of null hypothesis significance testing (NHST; I resisted the temptation to call it statistical hypothesis inference testing) to the point of meaninglessness and beyond. I argue herein that NHST has not only failed to support the advance of psychology as a science but also has seriously impeded it.   (Cohen 1994, p. 997)

At a basic level, the faulty probability logic of the NHST leads us astray. At another level, the hypothesis testing approach sets up a false dichotomy: if the p-value is significant, we accept the hypothesis; if it is not significant, we reject the hypothesis. This simplistic approach impedes progress in our knowledge, Cohen argues, because science just does not work this way: no single results proves or disproves a scientific hypothesis; rather, depending on the details of the study, we might be inclined to develop more or less confidence in that hypothesis based on individual study results. It is far from an all-or-nothing approach to decision-making, but rather a gradual approximation toward or away from a theory (see Chapter 16).

The Limits of Hypothesis-Testing

In sum, the concepts of p-values and statistical significance, though useful when used appropriately, are based on numerous assumptions which are not themselves based on statistics. In other words, there are some important features of these notions that are arbitrary and open to debate, not simply absolute truths to which we must pledge obedience. Even the formal logic of the hypothesis-testing approach is debatable.

This reality should be liberating to clinicians; statistics is not a field in which the numbers alone rule. Just like medicine, just like all human endeavor, statistics involve assumptions and beliefs. So, let us not be intimidated by statistics; nor should we devalue it. Unfortunately, most presentations of statistics ignore or whitewash the assumptions that are at the core of the primary axioms of statistics:

> The standard redaction of the Neyman-Pearson formulations found in elementary statistics textbooks tends to present hypothesis testing as a cut-and-dried procedure. Many purely arbitrary aspects of the methods are presented as immutable. While many of these arbitrary elements may not be appropriate for clinical research, the need that some medical scientists have to use 'correct' methods has enshrined an extremely rigid version of the Neyman-Pearson formulation. Nothing is acceptable unless the p-value cutoff is fixed in advanced and preserved by the statistical procedure. This was one reason why Fisher opposed the Neyman-Pearson formulation. He did not think that the use of p-values and significance tests should be subjected to such rigorous requirements . . .. Fisher suggested . . . that the final decision about what p-value should be significant should depend upon the circumstances. (Salsburg 2001a, pp. 278–9)

Forget P-Values: The Importance of Effect Sizes

In the preceding chapter, it was asserted that p-values are often misused in interpreting RCTs. They produce both false positive and false negative results. They should be used judiciously for the primary outcome of an RCT, and perhaps a few secondary outcomes, but that is all.

The solution otherwise is to forget about p-values and focus on effect sizes. Further, it is key to focus on absolute effect sizes, not just relative ones. This chapter will explain this concept.

Effect sizes tell you *how much* change was seen in a parameter. *How much* did the depression scale improve? p-Values only tell you that some change happened; there was some difference that cannot be explained by chance. But *how large* is that change? It could be tiny and still not have happened by chance (be statistically significant). It could be huge and not reach the p-value threshold of 0.05. Researchers need to pay attention to the effect size, the amount of change, and not just whether it happened by chance or not. A tiny change that is highly statistically significant can happen in a very large study; it is meaningless. A large change that is not statistically significant can happen in a small study; it could be very meaningful.

Forget about p-values. Turn to effect sizes.

And pay attention to absolute effect sizes, not just relative ones. Relative effect sizes are more well known: risk ratios (RR) or odds ratios (OR) are reported. These effect sizes, as explained later, reflect the relative frequency of an outcome in one group versus another. For instance, benefit is seen twice as frequently with drug vs placebo in depression (RR = 2). This difference might be highly statistically significant. But it may be meaningless if the absolute effect size, the actual amount of improvement with drug versus placebo, is small. The absolute effect size can be measured by change on a rating scale, such as number of points on a depression rating scale. If the benefit with drug is 15 points from beginning to end of the study, and benefit with placebo is 13 points from beginning to end of the study, then the difference is 2 points. This might be statistically significant, with a p-value below 0.05. It didn't happen by chance; but it is small, and clinically meaningless.

In fact, most antidepressant drugs have results as just described. They are published as "positive" because they are statistically significant, but the amount of improvement is small and not as clinically meaningful as many presume.

In short, statistical significance is not the same as clinically meaningful benefit – which is another way of saying that p-values are different from effect sizes.

So, let's understand what effect sizes are.

The Effect Estimation Approach

Effect sizes are central to what is called the "effect estimation" approach to statistics, just as p-values are central to the "hypothesis testing" approach to statistics. p-Values are legitimate if a study poses a hypothesis (x is better than placebo for depression) and then powers a study to a sample size to test that hypothesis. Effect estimation is legitimate everywhere else: one does not need a hypothesis, one simply describes the amount of benefit or harm with a drug in various outcomes.

The effect estimation approach breaks out the factors of effect size and precision (or variability of the data), providing more information, and in a more clearly presented form, than the hypothesis-testing approach. The main advantage of the effect estimation approach is that it does not require a pre-existing hypothesis (such as the null and alternative hypotheses), and thus we do not get into all the hazards of false negative and false positive results.

The best way to understand effect estimation, the alternative to hypothesis testing, is to appreciate the classic concept of a 2 × 2 table (Table 8.1). Here you have two groups: one that had the exposure (or treatment) and one that did not. Then you have two outcomes: yes or no (response or nonresponse; illness or nonillness).

Using a drug treatment for depression as an example, the effect size can simply be the percentage of responders: number who responded (a + c) ÷ number treated (a + b). Or it can be a relative risk: the likelihood of responding if given treatment would be a/a + b; the likelihood of responding if not given treatment would be c/c + d. So the relative likelihood of responding if given the treatment would be a/a + b ÷ c/c + d. This is often called the risk ratio and abbreviated as RR.

Another measure of relative risk is the odds ratio (OR), which mathematically equals ad/bc. The odds ratio is related to, but not the same as, the risk ratio. Odds are used to estimate probabilities, most commonly in settings of gambling. Probabilities can be said to range from 0% likelihood to 50 – 50 (meaning chance likelihood in either direction) to 100% absolute likelihood. Odds are defined as p/1 – p if p is the probability of an event. Thus, if the probability is 50% (or, colloquially, "50–50"), then the odds are 0.5/1 – 0.5 = 1. This is often expressed as "1 to 1." If the probability is absolutely likely, meaning 100%, then the odds are infinite: 1/1 – 1 = 1/0 = Infinity. Odds ratios approximate risk ratios; the only reason to distinguish them is that ORs are mathematically useful in regression models. When not using regression models, risk ratios are more intuitively straightforward.

The Effect Size

The effect estimation approach to statistics thus involves using effect sizes, like relative risks, as the main number of interest. The *effect size*, or the actual estimate of effect, is a number; this is whatever the number is – it may be a percentage (68% of patients were responders), an

Table 8.1 The epidemiological two-by-two table

	Outcome : yes	Outcome : no	
Exposure: yes	a	b	a + b
Exposure: no	c	d	c + d
	a + c	b + d	

actual number (the mean depression rating scale score was 12.4), or, quite commonly, a relative risk estimate: risk ratios (RR) or odds ratios (OR).

Many people use the term "effect size" to mean *standardized effect size*, which is a special kind of effect estimate. The standardized effect size, called Cohen's d, is the actual effect size described earlier (such as a mean number) divided by the standard deviation (the measure of variability). It produces a number that ranges from 0 to 1 or higher, and these numbers have meaning – but not unless one is familiar with the concept. Generally, it is said that an effect size of 0.4 or lower is small, 0.4 to 0.7 is medium, and more than 0.7 is large. Cohen's d is a useful measure of effect because it corrects for the variability of the sample, but it is less interpretable sometimes than the actual unadulterated effect size. For instance, if we report that the mean Hamilton Depression Rating Scale score (usually above 20 for severe depression) was 0.5 (zero being no symptoms) after treatment, we know that the effect size is large without needing to divide it by the standard deviation and get a Cohen's d greater than 1. Nonetheless, Cohen's d is especially useful in research using continuous measures of outcome (like psychiatric rating scales) and is commonly employed in experimental psychology research.

Another important estimate of effect, newer and more relevant to clinical psychiatry, is the *number needed to treat* (NNT) or the *number needed to harm* (NNH). This is a way of trying to give the effect estimate in a clinically meaningful way. Let us suppose that 60% of patients responded to a drug and 40% to placebo. One way to express the effect size is the risk ratio of 1.5 (60% divided by 40%). Another way of looking at it is that the difference between the two groups is 20% (60% – 40%). This is called the absolute risk reduction (ARR). The NNT is the reciprocal of the ARR, or 1/ARR: in this case, 1/0.20 = 5. Thus, for this kind of 20% difference between drug and placebo, clinically we can conclude that we need to treat 5 patients with the drug to get benefit in 1 of them. Again, certain standards are needed. Generally, it is viewed that a NNT of 5 or less is very large, 5–10 is large, 10–20 is moderate, above 20 is small, and more than 50 is likely meaningless.

A note of caution: This kind of abstract categorization of the size of the NNT is not exactly accurate. The NNT by itself may not fully capture whether an effect size is large or small. Some authors (e.g., Kraemer and Kupfer 2006) note, for instance, that the NNT for prevention of heart attack with aspirin is 130; the NNT for cyclosporine prevention of organ rejection is 6.3; and the NNT for effectiveness of psychotherapy (based on one review of the literature) is 3.1. Yet aspirin is widely recommended, cyclosporine is seen as a breakthrough, and psychotherapy is seen as "modest" in benefit. The explanation for these interpretations might be that the "hard" disease-modifying outcome of heart attack may justify a larger NNT with aspirin, as opposed to the "soft" merely symptomatic outcome of feeling better after psychotherapy. Aspirin is also cheap and easy to obtain, while psychotherapy is expensive and time-consuming (similarly, cyclosporine is expensive and associated with many medical risks).

NNT provides effect sizes, therefore, which need to be interpreted in the setting of the outcome being prevented and the costs and risks of the treatment being given.

The converse of the NNT is the number needed to harm (NNH), which is used when assessing side effects. Similar considerations apply to the NNH, and it is calculated in a similar way to the NNT. Thus, if an antipsychotic drug causes akathisia in 20% of patients versus 5% with placebo, then the ARR is 15% (20% – 5%), and the NNH is 1/0.15 = 6.7.

Clinical example: Absolute and relative effect sizes of antidepressant efficacy in "major depressive disorder"

Perhaps the most important clinical example of the central importance or understanding of absolute and relative effect sizes is the question of antidepressant efficacy in so-called major depressive disorder (MDD).

The key concept here is to understand both *absolute* and *relative* effect sizes.

The *absolute* effect size is simply how much the patient improves after antidepressant treatment compared to before treatment. So, if the patient starts with a Hamilton Depression Rating Scale score of 30, reflecting severe depression, and improves in 8 weeks to a score of 10, reflecting minimal depression, then the *absolute* effect size is a 20 point improvement.

The relative effect size is how much more the patient improves after antidepressant treatment compared to before placebo treatment versus how much the patient improves after placebo treatment compared to before placebo treatment. So, using the aforementioned antidepressant case of improvement in HDRS from 30 to 10 points in 8 weeks, a comparison would be made to a placebo-treated patient who improves in HDRS from 30 to 12 points at 8 weeks. Both patients improve markedly, but the difference in improvement between the groups is only 2 points on the HDRS scale (20 points for the antidepressant-treated patient versus 18 points for the placebo-treated patient). So, the *relative* effect size is a 2 point improvement.

What would we say about the case of these two patients? Keep in mind that a clinically meaningful effect size of benefit with the HDRS is set by government regulators as a 3 point difference between antidepressant improvement versus placebo improvement. In this case, there was a 2 point difference in improvement between the two treatments. So was the antidepressant effective or not?

From the standpoint of a relative effect size, and let's generalize so we are not referring to just two patients but to two treatment arms (one group treated with an antidepressant and another group treated with placebo), we would have to say that the antidepressant did not provide a clinically meaningful benefit over placebo. Or, to put it in other words, the antidepressant "didn't work."

But did it not work?

From the standpoint of absolute effect size, the antidepressant-treated group improved markedly from severe depression to minimal depression. A general definition of treatment response is a 50% improvement in symptoms, and the antidepressant group had 67% improvement in symptoms (from 30 points to 10 points). They clearly responded. They clearly improved. The problem is that the placebo group also improved markedly, so that the difference between the two groups is small. But that's a relative comparison. Getting back to the absolute effect, the antidepressant-treatment group improved. So it's not that the antidepressant "didn't work" in the sense that patients treated with it did not improve. The reality was that the antidepressant worked, and so did the placebo, so the improvement cannot be attributed to the pharmacological effect of the antidepressant.

This scenario is in fact the reality when it comes to the scientific evidence regarding antidepressant efficacy for acute depression in MDD.

About a decade ago, a classic meta-analysis examined all the available RCTs at that time assessing acute efficacy of modern antidepressants versus placebo for the acute depressive episode in MDD. The study became somewhat infamous, with the authors being interviewed in major media asserting that their review showed that antidepressants in generally did not have meaningful clinical efficacy. In other words, antidepressants "don't work."

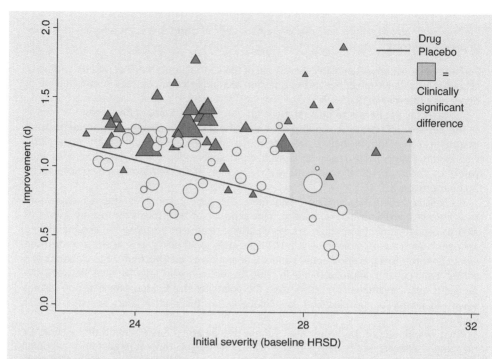

Figure 8.1 Antidepressants don't work?

In fact, their review was more complex. In the actual paper, Figure 8.1 is published. It compares the relative effect size of benefit, using Cohen's d, for antidepressants versus placebo, plotted by severity of depression. The general result is that there is almost no difference between antidepressant benefit vs placebo benefit for mild depression, some benefit but not much for moderate depression, and a larger, clinically meaningful benefit for severe depression.

To review Figure 8.1, Cohen's d is on the y axis, and the Hamilton Depression Rating Scale score is on the x axis. A Cohen's d score of near 1 or greater is a large absolute effect size of benefit. As can be seen, antidepressants show that large benefit in all levels of severity, with no change based on severity. In contrast, placebo shows a similar large benefit for mild depression, but it has a decreasing slope of benefit with severity, such that in marked depression, the difference between the two lines approximates a Cohen's d of about 0.5, which is the usual minimum standard for a clinically meaningful difference. Note, though, that even in severe depression, the absolute effect size for placebo alone is still about 0.7, which means that it still provides clinically meaningful benefit. Antidepressant is even higher, though, at around 1.2, hence the difference between the two lines of about 0.5.

This figure emphasizes why it is important to distinguish between absolute and relative effect sizes. Even in the worst-case scenario of mild depression, the clinical reality is not that antidepressants "don't work" but that everything works. Or, put another way, the benefit of antidepressants is large but it is not due to the pharmacological effects of antidepressants, since placebo worked just as well. In moderate depression there is some benefit, which might in fact be meaningful if analyzed differently, but for our purposes we can move on to severe depression and just note that there is clear benefit there with antidepressants. The authors' claim that antidepressants "don't work" was based on taking an average of these three subgroups: no benefit in mild depression, some benefit in moderate depression, clear benefit in severe depression. It all adds up to some benefit, but below the 0.5 Cohen's d threshold, and hence the misleading overall claim that the drugs don't work in general.

The same review reported the effect size also in terms of the scores on the Hamilton Depression Rating Scale. The mean difference between antidepressants and placebo was about 2 points on the HDRS. The threshold for a clinically meaningful difference has been set by the UK research agencies as 3 points on the HDRS, hence the claim that there was no clinically meaningful benefit with antidepressants over placebo. This claim needs to be revised, though, with the nuance of reporting effect sizes both in absolute terms, and in relative terms across severity subtypes. As noted, all patients improved in absolute HDRS scores. The 2–3 point figures have to do with the differences between antidepressant improvement and placebo improvement, but the overall improvement with both groups was much larger: around 10–15 points. Further, in severe depression, the difference between antidepressant and placebo was about 5 points, which is clinically meaningful.

As noted in Chapter 6, there is another aspect to this meta-analysis that is worth emphasizing, which has to do with why clinicians seem to think that antidepressants work so well while the RCTs suggest that they have small amounts of benefit overall. If we look at just the antidepressant group, without the placebo arm, which reflects clinical experience, clinicians and patients see that antidepressants have a large effect size of benefit, with Cohen's d above 1, no matter what the severity of depression. The antidepressant effect is large and consistent in all patients. The clinician who just believes his or her eyes would be justified in concluding that antidepressants work! And they work very well.

But that's why we need to do RCTs. The RCTs show you what causes the benefit seen with antidepressants. Adding the placebo arm, which can be known only by doing an RCT, not via clinical experience, tells the full story.

In mild depression, the benefit is not because of serotonin reuptake inhibition or any other pharmacological property of antidepressants. Rather, it has to do with causes captured in the placebo effect, such as natural history and psychological factors, as discussed in Chapter 9. In severe depression, most of the benefit still is nonpharmacological, but there some benefit is added by the pharmacological effects of antidepressants. This distinction, this ability to identify causes, is something which cannot be known in clinical experience or in clinical practice, but can be identified with RCTs. RCTs can inform clinicians about why they experience what they experience. RCTs provide information about scientific causation which clinical experience cannot provide.

Clinical example: Really, antidepressants work!

A second clinical example can be provided to show how important it is to measure absolute effect sizes, not just relative effect sizes. This example involves a recent, huge meta-analysis published in the most prestigious world medical journal, *The Lancet*, on the same topic: antidepressant efficacy in so-called MDD (Cipriani et al. 2018).

That meta-analysis seemed very clear: Antidepressants work. Really, they work! The study was cited extensively in the public media as showing that result, and the published paper in *The Lancet* clearly stated the conclusion that this definitive meta-analysis was proof of antidepressant efficacy in MDD.

The systematic review was an update on the 2008 study described earlier, and it seemed to come to an opposite conclusion. The 2008 meta-analysis concluded that antidepressants don't work; the 2018 meta-analysis concluded that they work. They used the same studies and the same methods; how could they come up with opposite conclusions? The implication in the *Lancet* paper was that the newer study was more definitive because it included newer studies, 522 RCTs in all, with a larger sample (more than 116,000 participants), with 21 different antidepressants. It was the last word.

But the last word was wrong, it turns out.

What did this prominent *Lancet* paper say? It conducted a standard meta-analysis of all available RCTs of antidepressants in MDD, published and unpublished (which is important; 52% of the included studies were unpublished), and, using this huge sample, it basically came up with a meta-analytic summary (see Chapter 12) of the *relative* risk of benefit with antidepressants versus placebo. The word "relative" is italicized to make the point about what the study did and what it did not do. If we see that the relative risk only is reported, the obvious second question is about *absolute* risk. We will get to that issue.

The relative risk reported is an odds ratio (OR). Recall that relative risk means the amount of benefit in one group divided by the amount of benefit in another group. So, a relative risk of 2.0 could mean that 40% responded with drugs versus 20% with placebo; or it could mean that 4% responded with drugs versus 2% with placebo. The absolute risk is the number that tells us whether we are dealing with large amounts of benefit, like 40% vs 20%, or small amounts of benefit, like 4% vs 2%.

The main report in the abstract was that "all antidepressants were more effective than placebo," with ORs ranging from 1.37 as the lowest figure for reboxetine to 2.13 as the highest figure for amitriptyline, as shown in Figure 8.2. Most agents had ORs of about 1.6 or

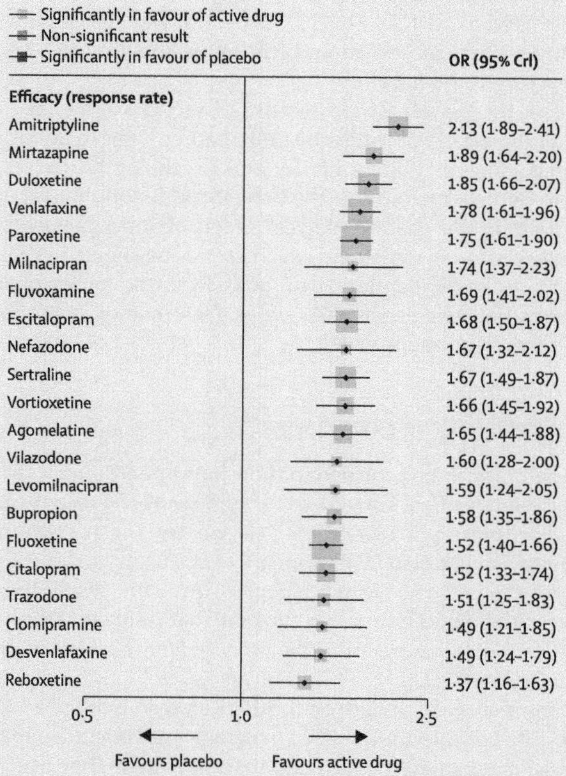

Figure 8.2 Lancet: Antidepressants work!

1.7. All outcomes were statistically significant, with confidence not including the null value of 1.

The main interpretation in the abstract was as follows: "All antidepressants were more efficacious than placebo in adults with major depressive disorder ....These results should serve evidence-based practice and inform patients, physicians, guideline developers, and policy makers on the relative merits of the different antidepressants" (Cipriani et al. 2018, p. 1357).

So what does this mean? The ORs were mostly about 1.6 to 1.7. That means that antidepressants were about 60–70% *relatively* more efficacious than placebo. But the conclusion didn't include the word "relatively"; it just said "were more efficacious." Let's remind ourselves what this means, using an OR of 2.0 as our standard. A two-fold benefit is a 100% relative improvement, so a 60–70% improvement is a bit less than a two-fold improvement. Again, that could mean almost 40% efficacy versus 20% efficacy, or it could mean 4% efficacy vs 2% efficacy. Which is it? In other words, what are the *absolute* effect sizes?

If one asks that question, there is nothing to be seen in the abstract. There is no report of any absolute effect size. There is nothing to be seen in the 10-page text of the published paper either. Ten pages in *The Lancet* is not a minor matter: that's prime publishing space. So, a lot was written in those ten pages about how the network meta-analysis was done (see chapter 12), about issues of potential bias in publication, and so on. There were five figures, mostly very colorful, one of which was very thorough and went into extensive detail with each drug about efficacy and tolerability outcomes. But it was all *relative* efficacy; there was no word about *absolute* efficacy.

The reader finds not a word in the results section about absolute effect sizes, like Cohen's d scores. In the discussion, on the first sentence of the second paragraph, one finds the only reference to possible absolute effect sizes in the published paper: "We found that all antidepressants included in the metaanalysis were more efficacious than placebo in adults with major depressive disorder and the summary effect sizes were mostly modest" (Cipriani et al. 2018, p. 1362). Nowhere else does the term "modest" appear in the paper in relation to effect sizes, nor is it mentioned again in the discussion or conclusions. The results turn out to be modest indeed, yet the paper was not presented as showing "modest" benefit, but rather that "antidepressants are more efficacious than placebo," with important policy and clinical implications, presumably supporting anti-depressant use.

So where are the data on the absolute effect sizes? Throughout the published paper, the authors refer to an online appendix. This kind of huge meta-analysis will produce a large amount of data, and these days such data can be made available to researchers in online form without the limitations of page limits in published journals. So, the reader in search of the absolute effect sizes has to leave the ten-page published paper, which received all the fanfare and which is all that almost everyone would read, and go to the online appendix.

The process is simple. By going to the article on the journal website, one clicks on the link for "supplementary material." Then one can download the entire online appendix as a PDF file. Once done, the reader finds that the online appendix is 290 pages long – essentially a book's worth of data for a large complex meta-analysis. Pages and pages of statistical software data outputs are found. The reader can be intimidated. But the table of contents is helpful. Under a section heading for "Results from network meta-analysis," one finds a subheading for "efficacy continuous" on page 150. The reader turns to page 150, smack dab in the middle of the nearly 300-page online appendix. There, the reader strikes gold, and sees Figure 8.3.

There it is – the holy grail of the search for an efficacy analysis. What does it show?

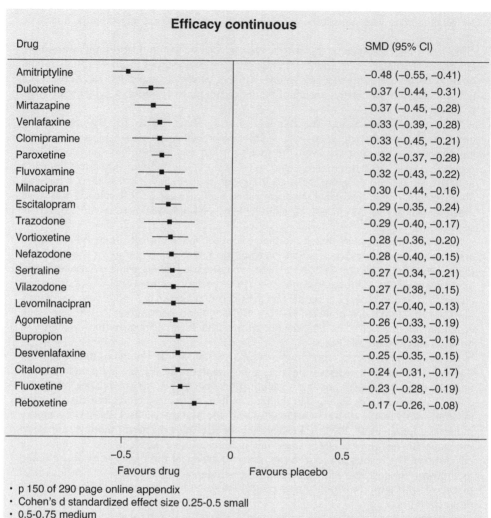

Figure 8.3 Lancet: Antidepressants don't work much

It provides standardized mean differences (SMDs), which reflect Cohen's d effect sizes. As seen in the figure, the Cohen's d effect sizes for almost all of the antidepressants are around 0.3 or so. Only one approximates 0.5, which is the usual cut-off for a clinically meaningful effect: amitriptyline, with a score of 0.48. The rest are notably lower than the threshold for clinically meaningful benefit. In fact, these results are basically the same as the earlier 2008 meta-analysis. Adding hundreds of RCTs and tens of thousands of new patients changed nothing.

Instead of showing that antidepressants work, this meta-analysis has the same result as the prior one: antidepressants have a small effect size of benefit over placebo, and it is not clinically meaningful. It is better than placebo, statistically significantly so, but that result only means it is not a chance finding. We know it's not a random result; it's believable. But what is the result? It's a small benefit, and not clinically meaningful.

This latter point is not made in the published paper, except in one sentence in the discussion where the efficacy is described as "modest," but nowhere else, especially in the abstract and conclusions, where an unqualified claim is made that "all antidepressants are more efficacious than placebo." While technically true, this is less than half the story. The amount of efficacy is minimal; that part is not stated.

Why did the authors not state the results more objectively? Why did they report the relative efficacy but not the absolute efficacy in the published paper? Why was the absolute efficacy buried in the middle of a nearly 300-page online appendix, without any emphasis or any interpretation? Why did the most prestigious medical journal publish such an article without asking these questions?

Understanding Placebo Effects

Many think that placebos are the most important aspect of clinical trials. This view is mistaken. Rather, as should be clear by now, randomization is the most important feature. Placebos usually go along with blinding, though some double-blind trials employ drugs only, without placebo. Many randomized studies, however, are perfectly valid without the use of any placebo. Thus, placebos are not the sine qua non of clinical trials; randomization is.

The principal rationale for using placebo is to control for the natural history of the illness. It is not because there are no active treatments available, and it is not because we want to maximize the drug-related effect size, though those features matter. The most important thing is to realize that most psychiatric illnesses resolve spontaneously, at least short-term, and thus placebo is needed to show that the use of drugs is associated with enough benefit over the natural history to outweigh the risks.

A common misconception is that benefits with placebo involve an inherent "placebo effect," which may consist of nonspecific psychosocial supportive factors, or possibly specific biological effects (Shepherd 1993). Such discussions often forget the effect of Nature (or God, if one prefers): the natural healing process. It is this natural history which is the essence of the placebo effect, although it might be augmented by nonspecific psychosocial supportive factors as well.

It is not even clear that the placebo effect is much of an effect, though many nonresearchers, especially psychotherapists, often assume that the placebo effect involves some relationship to supportive psychotherapy. A recent review of RCTs which had a placebo arm and a no-treatment arm – i.e., some patients who did not receive a placebo pill and also were not treated at all – found that placebo was not more effective than no treatment (Hrobjartsson and Gotzsche 2001).

Thus, many of our assumptions regarding placebo effects may need to be viewed as preliminary. I suggest that the main claim that can be best supported for now is that placebos reflect the natural history of the untreated illness.

Many critics think that placebos should *never* be used when a proven active treatment is available, viewing it as unethical to withhold such treatment (Moncrieff, Wessely, and Hardy 1998). The main argument against always comparing new drugs to active proven treatments is that the effect size will be smaller between those two groups, and thus larger numbers of people will be exposed to potentially ineffective or harmful drugs in RCTs. If fewer people can be studied with RCTs when placebo is used, and a drug turns out to be ineffective or harmful, then fewer people are exposed to risk (Emanuel and Miller 2001). In other words, drugs may simply not work. You need to have a placebo group to prove that they really do work; you can't just assume it. The continually instructive example of the RCT literature on antidepressants for so-called "MDD" explains this story.

Exploring Placebo Effects

As noted, a classic large meta-analysis of the Food and Drug Administration (FDA) database (which includes negative unpublished studies) argued that the benefits of drug over placebo involve a very small effect size when all RCTs are pooled in meta-analysis (Kirsch et al. 2008).

As mentioned previously, the results were more complicated, with large absolute benefit for both antidepressants and placebo. The difference between the two was small not because of poor antidepressant response, but because of large placebo response.

So That Explains That Large Placebo Response?

As stated, most people assume that the placebo response is just a psychological effect. This is only partly true. In conditions that are amenable to psychological influences, there may be a psychological component. These conditions would include diagnoses such as depression, pain syndromes, anxiety states, and psychosis. They would not include infectious diseases, cancers, or traumatic injury. In the latter states, psychological influences on outcomes are minimal, and the second important part of the placebo effect comes into play: the natural history of the illness.

Figure 9.1 presents natural history of illness and psychological effects as equal components of the placebo effect. But this varies depending on the illness. For most psychiatric illnesses, it is likely that natural history represents most of the placebo effect in most cases, while psychological influences are a notable but secondary factor.

Psychological Influences, Good and Bad

What are those psychological influences? They are not just about "expectancy effects," as is often stated. True, psychological expectancy matters: if the patient has a very positive attitude toward a pill, better results are obtained; if the patient has a very negative attitude toward a pill, worse results are obtained, which is called the "nocebo effect," or sometimes the "negative placebo effect." In other words, placebo effects aren't always for the better; they can also cause worse outcomes than the pharmacology of a treatment would cause by itself.

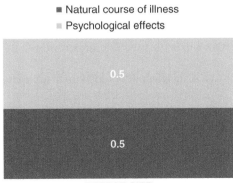

Figure 9.1 Placebo: Two main components

This nocebo effect is important in relation to side effects. If patients have a very negative disposition to taking a medication, they are likely to have many side effects from that medication, whether pharmacologically caused by the medication or not. Sometimes, patients search the list of identified side effects of a medication, and they tend to have those effects. Sometimes they have new and unusual ones. In any case, if a patient is highly reluctant to take medications, one reason not to push the matter is that many treatments are likely to fail because of nocebo-related side effects.

In a classic study (Myers, Cairns, and Singer 1987), the inclusion of gastrointestinal side effects in a list of potential adverse events in a consent form led to six times more reporting of such gastrointestinal side effects in comparison to a group who received the same consent form without inclusion of gastrointestinal side effects. This type of observation has been confirmed repeatedly.

The Psychological Effects of Pill-Giving Often Are Harmful, Not Beneficial

There is another aspect, though: the clinician–patient relationship, often referred to as the therapeutic alliance. This part of the placebo effect is relevant not only to pill placebos but also to nonpill placebos, such as psychotherapies. Even manualized, highly empirical psychotherapies, such as cognitive behavioral therapy (CBT), have a placebo effect based on the interpersonal relationship between the therapist and the client. The leader of modern CBT, Aaron Beck, was a kindly, pleasant gentleman. His kindness, and not the technical method of CBT, likely explained some of his results. Beck himself often admitted as much, including in his final papers:

> In addition to identifying the primary problem and working to rewire maladaptive beliefs and biases into more adaptive ones, another key factor in the success of any of the adaptations of cognitive therapy is the working relationship with the therapist. In the most severe problems, such as personality disorders – borderline personality disorder and schizophrenia, for example – the forging of the connection with the patient involves a kind of partnership or comradeship in many cases.   (Beck 2019, p. 19)

I recall that decades ago, when I gave a lecture on mood stabilizers to an audience of community psychiatrists in Quebec, one of them commented afterwards about all the treatment benefits I had described. "You talked about the medications as mood stabilizers," he said. "I think *you're* the mood stabilizer," he added, pointing at me. "I think I'm the mood stabilizer," he finished, touching his chest. At the time, I thought his comments a bit exaggerated, but with time I've grown more and more convinced of his wisdom.

A drug effect is never just a drug effect. It is added to or subtracted from by the clinician–patient relationship.

In fact, the therapeutic alliance has been reported to represent most of the benefit seen with psychotherapy treatments of all kinds, irrespective of specific methods such as CBT as opposed to Freudian approaches (Martin, Garske, and Davis 2000; Fluckiger et al. 2018; Fluckiger et al. 2012). A National Institute of Mental Health treatment of depression study that included both CBT and tricyclic antidepressants versus placebo found that the therapeutic alliance also influenced the drug outcomes, with about 21% of the overall benefit attributed to the therapeutic alliance (Krupnick et al. 1996).

Doctors and clinicians long have been taught the importance of the relationship with the patient. Traditionally, it was called "bedside manner"; now, the "therapeutic alliance." It is a major part of the psychological aspect of placebo effects.

Natural History

The second aspect of the placebo effect is that the inert pill is a stand-in for absence of treatment – in other words, the natural history of the illness. This aspect of the placebo effect applies to all conditions, whether psychologically malleable or not. It would apply to depression, pain, anxiety, and psychosis, but also to infectious disease, cancers, traumatic injuries, and any medical illness of any kind. It is this part of the placebo effect that is universal, whereas psychological impacts are more variable. That's because all diseases have a natural history, but not all diseases can be influenced equally by psychological influences.

This aspect of the placebo effect is very important to understand in psychiatric illnesses in particular. Contrary to popular belief, most psychiatric illnesses, excluding a few such as schizophrenia, are not very severe, at least in the sense of never going away. Most psychiatric states go away on their own. They may be quite painful, they may be debilitating, they may be horrible in many ways; but they end on their own, without any intervention at all. That's why psychiatry functioned as a profession for a century before the first effective medications were developed in the mid-twentieth century. Suicide is a terrible outcome, but it is relatively uncommon. If someone has a severe period of depression, it has a beginning and an end. We speak of "episodes" of depression or mania or psychosis because they always end. The only chronic condition which persists once the disease has begun is schizophrenia. Otherwise, almost all major psychiatric states of pathology are episodic: they have a beginning and an end, without any treatment.

This aspect of most psychiatric states can be restated by saying that the natural history is characterized by spontaneous recovery. Of course, this recovery doesn't mean that patients never have any symptoms ever again. Episodes tend to recur in the future. But for the current episode, it ends; it's over. Long-term studies would have lower placebo effects since recurrence is extremely common, but short-term studies would have a massive placebo effect due to the usual natural recovery of the acute episode. And most studies of psychiatric treatments are short term.

More than a century of pretreatment-era psychiatric research, dating from the 1960s back to Kraepelin and others in the nineteenth century, provides a large database on the natural history of psychiatric illnesses. For severe depressive episodes in nonbipolar subjects, one could summarize this large literature by saying that the average episode lasts 6–12 months. For bipolar depression, the average episode lasts 3–6 months. For manic episodes, the average episode lasts 2–4 months. Typically, before patients begin treatment trials, they will have experienced their mood state for weeks to months.

In a study of MDD, if we take one month as a baseline period of mood symptoms, then a study of depression that lasts 8 weeks would represent 3 months of depression for the placebo group. Since the average improvement is 6–12 months, this 3 month duration likely would include a small recovery by natural history. However, if some of the included patients had been depressed for 2–4 months before the study began, then they would be 4–6 months into the natural course of their depressive episodes, and they would have higher natural history recovery rates that would be captured in the placebo response.

Much higher placebo response rates will be seen in bipolar depression studies because of the shorter natural duration of episodes. If we take one month as a baseline period of mood symptoms, then a study of bipolar depression that lasts 8 weeks would represent 3 months of depression for the placebo group. Since the average improvement is 3–6 months, this 3 month duration likely would include a large amount of recovery by natural history. If some of the included patients had been depressed for 2–4 months before the study began, then they would be 4–6 months into the natural course of their depressive episodes, and almost all patients in the placebo group would recover based on natural history alone. This fact is why bipolar depression trials, typically 6 weeks long, should be shorter than unipolar depression trials, typically 8 weeks long. A good example is provided by RCTs of aripiprazole in bipolar depression (Marcus et al. 2008), which were 8 weeks long. At 4 and 6 weeks, aripiprazole was more effective than placebo, but not at 8 weeks. The placebo effect increased between 6 and 8 weeks.

Since 8 weeks was the primary outcome, the makers of aripripazole were not able to get FDA indications for that drug for bipolar depression. When they conducted studies of the same agent in MDD lasting 8 weeks, they were able to show benefit over placebo and received FDA indication. Later trials with other agents in bipolar depression, such as quetiapine, were 6 weeks long and showed benefit over placebo.

Since mania is even briefer, shorter studies are required to show benefit over placebo. Mania trials only are three weeks in duration.

Exploring Natural History: Placebo vs Nonplacebo Nontreatment

Can one directly measure the effect of natural history? After all, if placebo consists of part psychological influences and part natural history, how can one know how much of each kind is present? It turns out that natural history can be measured if there is a third group besides treatment versus placebo: a nonplacebo nontreatment arm. This last arm can be a waiting list control group, or a group which does not receive an active pill but also receives no inert pill. In such patients, there is no psychological influence because there is no interaction with clinicians and there is no ingestion of a pill of any kind.

There have been about half a dozen such studies in antidepressant treatment trials of MDD. As can be seen in Figure 9.2, in depressed patients who were untreated and received no placebo but simply were on a waiting list, an absolute effect size of improvement of Cohen's d of 0.5 was seen, which is a clinically meaningful benefit. This change represented about a 4 point absolute improvement in standard depression ratings scales. Thus, if a patient began with a depression score of 22, the improvement would be to about 18. The patient would remain notably depressed, but less so after 8 weeks of gradual natural improvement.

If we imagine a patient who might improve by 10 points on a standard depression rating scale, like the MADRS, from 25 at start to 15 at 8 weeks, then almost half of that improvement is attributable solely to the natural history of recovery without introducing any psychological influences at all, such as the clinician–patient relationship or the patient's own psychological expectations for treatment.

We can now put all these factors together to better understand the individual impact of the three influences of recovery in treatment studies: natural history (untreated recovery in

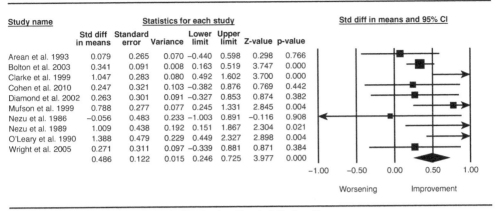

Study name	Statistics for each study								Std diff in means and 95% CI
	Std diff in means	Standard error	Variance	Lower limit	Upper limit	Z-value	p-value		
Arean et al. 1993	0.079	0.265	0.070	−0.440	0.598	0.298	0.766		
Bolton et al. 2003	0.341	0.091	0.008	0.163	0.519	3.747	0.000		
Clarke et al. 1999	1.047	0.283	0.080	0.492	1.602	3.700	0.000		
Cohen et al. 2010	0.247	0.321	0.103	−0.382	0.876	0.769	0.442		
Diamond et al. 2002	0.263	0.301	0.091	−0.327	0.853	0.874	0.382		
Mufson et al. 1999	0.788	0.277	0.077	0.245	1.331	2.845	0.004		
Nezu et al. 1986	−0.056	0.483	0.233	−1.003	0.891	−0.116	0.908		
Nezu et al. 1989	1.009	0.438	0.192	0.151	1.867	2.304	0.021		
O'Leary et al. 1990	1.388	0.479	0.229	0.449	2.327	2.898	0.004		
Wright et al. 2005	0.271	0.311	0.097	−0.339	0.881	0.871	0.384		
	0.486	0.122	0.015	0.246	0.725	3.977	0.000		

−1.00   −0.50   0.00   0.50   1.00

Worsening   Improvement

Absolute benefit, not relative benefit

How much did they improve after 10 weeks? Mean improvement in HDRS = 4 points.

Standardized effect size = 0.486

10 trials had a mean sample size of 32.3 ± 51.6 patients, duration of 10.0 ± 3.7 weeks, and dropout rate of 18.6% ± 17.1%.

Figure 9.2 Natural course: What if you do nothing? Source: Rutherford et al. 2012

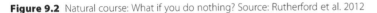

episodic illness), psychological influences (clinician–patient relationship, psychological expectations), and the treatment (drug or psychotherapy).

The Floor Effect

Returning to the meta-analysis of antidepressant clinical trials of MDD (Kirsch et al. 2008), we observed that the overall small effect size was a misleading average of differing results based on severity of depression. When looking at the severely depressed population, it appears that there is a larger beneficial effect size of antidepressants over placebo because of a lower placebo response; in contrast, the antidepressant drug effect was stable whether severity was mild, moderate, or severe. It was the placebo effect which declined (Figure 8.1).

So, we see the interplay of pharmacological effect of the drug and placebo effect, differing based on severity of illness. It is a well-known aspect of the placebo effect that it is higher for milder symptoms and lower for more severe symptoms. This relationship can be understood by thinking of the two major components of the placebo effect: psychological expectancy and natural history. If someone has mild symptoms, a good psychological relationship with the clinician, or a small improvement by natural history, this can improve symptoms sufficiently to lead to feeling much better. On the other hand, a similar amount of benefit for severe symptoms would not lead to enough benefit in the end.

This difference based on severity is called a *floor effect*: you can never get better than a score of zero on a symptom rating scale. So the closer you begin to zero, the easier it will be to feel better.

Look at Figure 9.3 to understand this effect.

With standard depression rating scales, a score of 20 and above tends to reflect a full clinical depressive episode; 50% improvement reflects a clinical response, with scores falling by one-half. If someone has mild depression, with a baseline score of 20 on a depression rating scale, then clinical response would be a 10-point improvement – 50% of 20 – with an

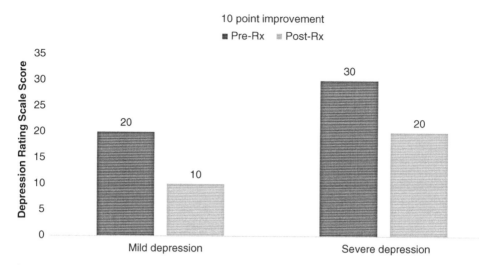

Figure 9.3 Floor effect: Less room for improvement with mild depression

endpoint score of 10. A score of 10 on standard depression rating scales reflects mild symptoms, below the threshold for a full episode.

But if someone has severe depression, with a baseline score of 30 on a depression rating scale, then the same absolute improvement of 10 points would lead to an endpoint score of 20, meaning that the patient improved somewhat but remains clinically depressed. By percentage improvement, this 10 point change would only be a 33% improvement from baseline.

So, we see the same absolute improvement in both cases – 10 points – but different relative improvements: 50% versus 33%. In the case of mild depression, the patient goes from feeling depressed to having minimal depressive symptoms; in the case of severe depression, the patient goes from being very depressed to being less symptomatic but still clinically depressed.

The absolute improvement is the same in both cases. The difference is the floor effect. In mild depression, the patient needed to improve less to notice more benefit. In severe depression, there is more room for improvement and a larger benefit is needed to obtain it.

So, getting back to the placebo effect, if patients have mild symptoms, a small absolute improvement can have an important clinical effect. This effect can happen either with psychological influences or with natural history.

Synthesis

Putting it all together, as shown previously, Figure 9.4 demonstrates the three influences on antidepressant response: natural history, psychological influences, and drug pharmacology.

The figure uses the data from the foregoing meta-analysis, and the literature on natural history reviewed previously, using Cohen's d effect sizes. The overall summary result is a difference between antidepressant and placebo of d = 0.3, which is below the threshold of a clinically meaningful difference of 0.5. However, when we examine absolute effect sizes, we see that the overall effect size of antidepressants was 1.5 versus 1.2 for placebo, hence the 0.3

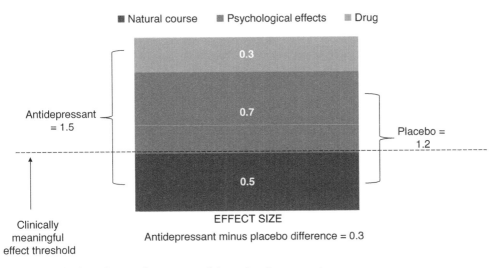

Figure 9.4 Absolute effect size for treatment of depression: 3 components

relative difference. We know from the natural history systematic review that the effect of natural recovery is an effect size of 0.5. We also know that the pharmacological effect size of drug over placebo is 0.3, as just described. Since the total effect size of the drug is 1.5, then subtracting natural history (0.5) and placebo (0.3) leaves a remaining effect size of 0.7, which can be attributed to the psychological factor of placebo response.

Understanding the two components of the placebo effect allows us to understand the overall real pharmacological impact of antidepressants for depressive states. Patients improve markedly (absolute Cohen's d = 1.5), but about half of that improvement has to do with psychological influences (the clinician–patient relationship, patient expectations), a third has to do with the natural course of the illness leading to recovery, and the smallest part (about one-fifth of the effect) has to do with the pharmacological effects of the drugs.

Severity influences these interpretations, as shown in Figures 9.5 and 9.6.

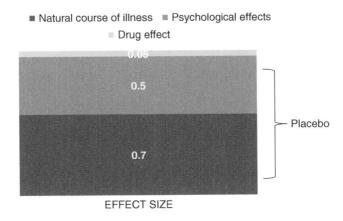

Figure 9.5 Mild depression: Drug plus placebo components

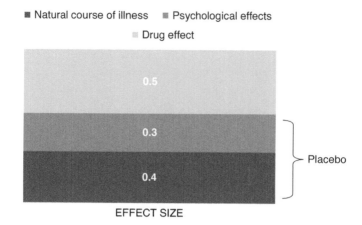

Figure 9.6 Severe depression: Drug plus placebo components

In mild depression, drug effect is almost nothing (0.05), while psychological influences represent 2/3 of benefit (0.95), and natural history 1/3 of benefit (0.5). In severe depression, drug effect is larger and all three influences are equally effective at d = 0.5.

In all cases, we see that drug effect is never larger than natural history, and the most fluctuating influence is the psychological component.

Understanding Confidence Intervals

Jerzy Neyman, who developed the basic structure of hypothesis-testing statistics, also advanced the alternative approach of effect estimation with the concept of *confidence intervals* in 1934.

The rationale for confidence intervals stems from the fact that we are dealing with probabilities in statistics and in all medical research. We observe something – say, a 45.9% response rate with drug Y. Is the *real* value 45.9%, rather than 45.6%, or 46.3%? How much *confidence* do we have in the number we observe? In traditional statistics, the view is that there is a real number that we are trying to discover (let's say that God, who knows all, knows that the real response rate with drug Y is 46.1%). Our observed number is a *statistic*, an estimate of the real number. (Fisher had defined the word statistic "as a number that is derived from the observed measurements and that estimates a parameter of the distribution"; Salsburg 2001a, p. 89.) But we need to have some sense of how plausible our statistic is, how well it reflects the likely real number. The concept of confidence intervals (CIs) as developed by Neyman was not itself a probability; this was not just another variation of p-values. Rather, Neyman saw it as a conceptual construct that helped us appreciate how well our observations have approached reality. As Salsburg puts it:

> the confidence interval has to be viewed not in terms of each conclusion but as a process. In the long run, the statistician who always computes 95 percent confidence intervals will find that the true value of the parameter lies within the computed interval 95 percent of the time. Note that, to Neyman, the probability associated with the confidence interval was not the probability that we are correct. It was the frequency of correct statements that a statistician who uses his method will make in the long run. It says nothing about how "accurate" the current estimate is. (Salsburg 2001a, p. 123)

We can, therefore, make the following statements: *Confidence intervals* can be defined as *the range of plausible values* for the effect size. Another way of putting this is that it is *the likelihood that the real value for the variable would be captured in 95% of trials*. Or, alternatively, *if the study was repeated over and over again, the observed results would fall within the confidence intervals 95% of the time.* (More formally defined, the CI is: "The interval computed from sample data that has a given probability that the unknown parameter . . . is contained within the interval"; Dawson and Trapp 2001, p. 335.)

Confidence intervals use a theoretical computation that involves the mean and the standard deviation, or variability, of the distribution. This can be stated as follows: The confidence interval for a mean is the observed mean ± (confidence coefficient) × the variability of the mean. The CI uses mathematical formulae similar to what are used to calculate p-values (each extreme is computed at 1.96 standard deviations from the mean in a normal distribution), and thus the 95% limit of a CI is equivalent to a p-value = 0.05. This is why CIs can give the same information as p-values, but CIs also give much more: the probability of the observed findings when compared to the computed normal distribution.

The CI is *not* the probability of detecting the true parameter. It does not mean that you have a 95% probability of having detected the true value of the variable. The true value has either been detected or not; we do not know whether it has fallen within our confidence intervals. The CIs instead reflect the likelihood of such being the case with repeated testing.

Another way of relating CIs to hypothesis testing is as follows: A hypothesis test tells us whether the observed data are consistent with the NH. A confidence interval tells us which hypotheses are consistent with the data. Another way of putting this is that the p-value gives you a yes or no answer: Are the data highly likely (meaning p > 0.05) to have been observed by chance? (Or, alternatively, are we highly likely to mistakenly reject the NH by chance?) Yes or No? The CIs give you more information: they provide actual effect size (which p-values do not) and (like p-values) they provide an estimate of precision (which p-values do not: How likely are the observed means to differ if we are to repeat the study?). Since the information provided by a p-value of 0.05 is the same as what is provided by a confidence interval of 95%, there is no need to provide p-values when confidence intervals are used (although researchers routinely do so, perhaps because they think that readers cannot interpret CIs). Or, put another way, CIs provide all the information one finds in p-values, *and more*; hence, the relevance of the proposal, somewhat serious, that p-values should be abolished altogether in favor of CIs (Lang, Rothman, and Cann 1998).

Clinical example: The antidepressants and suicide controversy

For almost two decades, debates have persisted around the impact of standard antidepressants on suicidality in children and young adults. The clinical implications of any potential suicidal harm also have been discussed, without a clear consensus in the clinical community. Prior analyses have not used quantitative risk–benefit analyses including absolute harm or risk rates. In this chapter, that analysis is conducted and demonstrates that the clinical implications are not supportive of antidepressant use, nor do they demonstrate a large absolute risk as a reason to avoid treatment.

Early Views

When the FDA issued its first black box warning regarding antidepressants and suicidality in children (Hammad, Laughren, and Racoosin 2006), two opposite views hardened immediately: Critics of psychiatric drugs saw antidepressants as harmful and held that they should be avoided in children (Jureidini et al. 2004), while the mainstream of the psychiatric profession, unwilling to admit any validity to the claim of a link to suicidality, professed the reverse (Isacsson and Rich 2014). An example of the latter was a report by a task force of the American College of Neuropsychopharmacology (ACNP) (Mann et al. 2006). By pooling different studies with each serotonin reuptake inhibitor (SRI) separately, and showing that each of those agents did not reach statistical significance in showing a link with suicide attempts, the ACNP task force claimed that there was *no evidence at all* of such a link, ignoring the fact that when added together to have sufficient sample size, as in the FDA meta-analysis, such a relationship was found. In its meta-analysis, the FDA was able to demonstrate not only statistical significance, but also a concerning effect size of about a two-fold increased risk of suicidality (suicide attempts or increased suicidal ideation) with SRIs over placebo (RR = 1.95, 95% CIs 1.28, 2.98) (Hammad, Laughren, and Racoosin 2006).

Absolute Effect Size As the Solution

These debates about the clinical relevance of the FDA finding could have been solved more quickly if the relative effect sizes reported earlier were augmented with discussion of absolute effect sizes. Here, the concept of a number needed to harm (NNH) becomes useful. In the FDA meta-analysis, the absolute difference between placebo and SRIs was 0.1%. This is a real risk, but obviously a small one absolutely, which is seen when converted to NNH (1 / 0.01) = 100. Thus, of every 100 patients treated with antidepressants, 1 patient would make a suicide attempt attributable to them. One could then compare this risk, with presumed benefit.

This is the proper way to analyze such data: not by relying on anecdote to claim massive harm, nor by misusing p-values to claim no harm at all. Descriptive statistics tell the true story: there is harm, but it is small. Then, the art of medicine takes over – what William Osler called the art of balancing probabilities. The benefits of antidepressants would then need to be weighed against this small, but real, risk.

The Treatment of Adolescent Depression Study

In moving to that kind of risk–benefit analysis, it would also be helpful to look at other randomized trials besides the pharmaceutical industry studies used in the FDA review. As many critics point out, there were no completed suicides in the FDA meta-analysis. This fact is not surprising since pharmaceutical trials are carefully conducted to exclude patients with active or severe suicidal ideation or recent suicide attempts. In the typical 8-week period of study, one would not expect completed suicides; they occur rarely if at all. Instead, it is remarkable that there was detection of an increase in suicide attempts and that suicidal ideation was seen in this highly selected nonsuicidal population.

Nonetheless, as with any topic, the best study is one which is designed to study the question itself. The pharmaceutical industry antidepressant clinical trials were not designed to assess suicidality; they were powered and designed to test clinical efficacy for depressive symptoms as a whole. The low frequency of increased suicidality was such that those studies, one by one, also were too small to definitively prove or disprove an association – hence the need for meta-analysis.

Another approach was to conduct a larger RCT to try to answer the question, with a specific plan to look at suicidality as a secondary outcome (unlike all the studies in the FDA database). This led to the National Institute of Mental Health (NIMH)-sponsored Treatment of Adolescent Depression Study (TADS) (March et al. 2004). Yet even there, where no pharmaceutical influence existed based on funding, the investigators appear to underreport the suicidal risks of fluoxetine by overreliance on p-value-based hypothesis-testing methods.

In that study, 479 adolescents were double-blind randomized in a factorial design to fluoxetine vs CBT vs both vs neither. Response rates were 61% vs 43% vs 71% vs 35%, respectively, with differences being statistically significant. Clinically significant suicidality was present in 29% of children at baseline (more than in most previous studies, which is good because it provides a larger number of outcomes for assessment), and worsening suicidal ideation or a suicide attempt was defined as the secondary outcome of "suicide related adverse events." (No completed suicides occurred in 12 weeks of treatment.) A total of 7 suicide attempts were made, 6 of which were on fluoxetine. In the abstract, the investigators reported improvement in suicidality in all four groups, but without commenting on the differential worsening in the fluoxetine group. The text reported 5.5% (24) suicide-related adverse events, but it did not report the results with RR and CIs. When analyzed that way, one sees the following risk of worsened suicidality: with fluoxetine, RR 1.77 [0.76, 4.15]; with CBT, RR 0.85 [0.37, 1.94]. The paper speculates about possible protective benefits with CBT for suicidality, even though the CIs are too wide to infer much probability of such benefit. In contrast, the apparent increase in suicidal risk with fluoxetine, which appears more probable based on the CIs than in the CBT effect, is not discussed in as much detail. The low suicide attempt rate (1.6%, n = 7) is reported, but the overwhelming prevalence with fluoxetine use is not. Using effect estimate methods, the risk of suicide attempts with fluoxetine is RR 6.19 [0.75, 51.0]. Due to the low frequency, this risk is not statistically significant. But hypothesis testing methods are inappropriate here; use of effect estimation shows a large 6-fold risk, which is probably present, and which could be as high as 51-fold.

Hypothesis-testing methods, biased toward the null hypothesis, tell one story; effect estimation methods, less biased and more neutral, tell another. For side effects in general, especially for infrequent ones like suicidality, the effect estimation stories are closer to reality.

An Oslerian Approach to Antidepressants and Suicide

Recalling Osler's dictum that the art of medicine is the art of balancing probabilities, we can conclude that the antidepressant/suicide controversy is not a question of yes or no, but rather of whether there is a risk, quantifying that risk, and then weighing that risk against the benefits.

This effort has not been made systematically, but one researcher made a start in a letter to the editor of *JAMA* commenting on the TADS study (Carroll 2004). Carroll noted that the NNH for suicide-related averse events in the TADS study was 34 (6.9% with fluoxetine versus 4.0% without it). The NNH for suicide attempts was 43 (2.8% with fluoxetine versus 0.45% without it). In contrast, the benefit seen with improvement of depression was more notable; the NNT for fluoxetine was 3.7.

So, about 4 patients need to be treated to improve depression in 1 of them, while a suicide attempt due to fluoxetine will only occur after 43 patients are treated. This would seem to favor the drug, but we are really comparing apples and oranges: improving depression is fine, but how many deaths due to suicide from the drug are we willing to accept?

One has to now bring in other probabilities besides the actual data from the study (an approach related to Bayesian statistics): Epidemiological studies indicate that about 8% of suicide attempts end in death (Conner, Azrael, and Miller 2019). Thus, with a NNH for suicide attempts of 43, the NNH for completed suicide would be 537 (43 divided by 0.08; see Table 10.1). This would seem to be a very small risk, but it is a serious outcome. Can we balance it by an estimate of prevention of suicide?

A conservative estimate of lifetime suicide in major depressive disorder (MDD) is 3.4% (Blair-West et al. 1999). More adolescents and young adults commit suicide than older adults, although the relative rates are higher in the older population. About one-half of all suicides in patients with MDD happened before age 44, but the exact number that happen before age 18 is not well established (Bachmann 2018). We do know that young adults have a higher rate than adolescents, who have a higher rate than younger children. If we assume

Table 10.1 Risk–benefit analysis of antidepressant prevention vs causation of completed suicide in children and adolescents

Analysis	NNT (prevention of suicide)*	NNH (causation of suicide)	Likelihood of help to harm (1/NNT/NNH)
FDA	870	1,250	1.44
TADS	870	535	0.61

* TADS data for prevention was used for both analyses.

that about 25% of suicides in MDD before age 44 will happen in childhood or adolescence, then the overall rate will be around 0.0425% of all children and adolescents with MDD (3.4% × 0.5 × 0.25). This produces a NNT for prevention of suicide with fluoxetine, based on the TADS data, of 870 (3.7 divided by 0.00425; see Table 10.1).

We could also do the same kind of analysis using the FDA database cited previously, which found an NNH for suicide attempts of 100 (higher than the TADS study) (Hammad, Laughren, and Racoosin 2006). If 8% of those patients complete suicide, then the NNH for completed suicide is 1,250 (100 divided by 0.08; see in Table 10.1).

So, we save one life out of every 870 that we treat, and we lose one life out of every 535, or possibly every 1,250 patients. As shown in Table 10.1, there seems to be more evidence of possible harm using the TADS rather than using the FDA database, but in both cases the relative benefit or harm is close to the null value of one. Given the small absolute frequencies, and applying Osler's dictum about the art of medicine meaning balancing probabilities, the risk is small either way. It is also possible that the actual suicide rates used earlier are too conservative, and that antidepressants might have somewhat more preventive benefit than suggested herein, but even with more benefit their relative benefit would still be far above an NNT of 100, which is generally consider minimal.

Overall, then antidepressants have minimal benefits, and minimal risks, at least in general terms, in relation to suicide in children and adolescents.

LHH is interpreted as patients being 0.61 to 1.44 times more likely to be helped than harmed in prevention of suicide.

Lessons Learned

At some level, the controversy about antidepressants and suicide had to do with mistaken abuse of hypothesis testing statistics. The proponents of the association argued that anecdotes were real, and were not refuted by the RCTs. They were correct. Their opponents claimed that the amount of risk shown in RCTs was small. They were correct. Both sides erred when they claimed their view was absolutely correct: Based on anecdote, one side wanted to view antidepressants as dangerous in general; based on statistical nonsignificance, the other side wanted to argue there was no effect at all.

Both groups had no adequate comprehension of science, medical statistics, or evidence-based medicine. When effect estimation methods are applied, and the concept of confidence intervals was used instead of p-values, one observes that there appears to be a real risk of suicide with antidepressants, but that risk is small and equal to or less than the probable benefit of prevention of suicide with such agents.

Observational Studies

Cohort Studies

The standard use of effect estimation statistics is in prospective cohort studies. In this case the exposure occurs before the outcome. The main advantages of the prospective cohort study are that researchers do not bias their observations since they state their hypotheses before the outcomes have occurred; also, researchers usually collect the outcomes systematically in such studies. Thus, although the data are still observational and not randomized, the regression analysis that later follows can use a rich dataset in which many of the relevant confounding variables are fully and accurately collected.

Classic examples of prospective cohort studies in medicine are the Framingham Heart Study and the Nurses Health Study, both of which have been ongoing now for decades and which are rich sources of useful knowledge about cardiovascular disease. An example of a psychiatric cohort study, conducted for five years, was the Systematic Treatment Enhancement Program for Bipolar Disorder (STEP-BD) project.

Chart Reviews: Pros and Cons

Prospective cohort studies are expensive and time-consuming. The five-year STEP-BD project cost about $20 million. There are many, many more important medical questions that need to be answered than can be approached either by RCTs or prospective cohort studies. Hence, we are forced to rely, for some questions and at some phases of the scientific research process, on retrospective cohort studies. Here the outcomes have already occurred, and thus there is more liability to bias on the part of researchers looking for the causes that may have led to those outcomes.

A classic example of a retrospective cohort study is the case-control paradigm. In this kind of study, cases with an outcome (e.g., lung cancer) are compared with controls who do not have the outcome (no lung cancer). The two groups are then compared on an exposure (e.g., rates of cigarette smoking). The important issue is to try to match the case and control groups as much as is feasible on all possible factors except for the experimental variable of interest. This is usually technically infeasible beyond a few basic features such as age, gender, ethnicity, and similar variables. The risk of confounding bias is very high. Regression analysis can help reduce confounding bias in a large enough sample, but one is often faced with a lack of adequate data previously collected on many relevant confounding variables.

All these limitations given, it is still relevant that retrospective cohort studies are important sources of scientific evidence and that they are often correct. For instance, the relationship between cigarette smoking and lung cancer was almost completely established in the 1950s and 1960s based on retrospective case-control studies, even without any statistical regression analysis (which had not yet been developed).

Despite a long period of criticism of those data by skeptics, those case-control results have stood up to the test of other, better-designed studies and analyses.

Nonetheless, the limitations of retrospective cohort study deserve some examination.

Limitations of Retrospective Observational Studies

One of these limitations, especially relevant for psychiatric research, is *recall bias*: the fact that people have poor memories for their medical history. In one study, patients were asked to recall their past treatments with antidepressants for up to five years; these recollections were then compared to the actual documented treatments kept by the same investigators in their patient charts. The researchers found that patients recalled 80% of treatments received in the prior year, which may not seem bad; but by five years they only recalled 67% of treatments received (Posternak and Zimmerman 2003). Since some chart reviews extend back decades, we can expect that we are only getting about half the story if we rely mainly on a patient's self-report. While this is a problem, there is also a reality: prospective studies lasting decades in duration will not be available for most of the medical questions that we need to answer. So again, using *real* (not ivory-tower) EBM: *some data, any data, properly analyzed, are better than no data.* I would view this glass as half full, and take the information available in chart reviews, with the appropriate level of caution; I would not, as many academics do, see it as half empty and thus reject such studies as worthless.

Another example of recall bias relates to diagnosis. A major depressive episode is usually painful and patients know they are sick: they do not lack insight into depression. Thus, one would expect reasonably good recall of having experienced severe depression in the past. In a study, however, researchers interviewed 45 patients who had been hospitalized 25 years earlier for a major depressive episode (Andrews et al. 1999). Twenty-five years later, 70% recalled being depressed and only 52% were able to give adequate detail for researchers to be able to fully identify sufficient criteria to meet the severity of a full major depressive episode. So, even with hospitalized depression, 30% of patients do not recall the symptoms at all decades later, and only 50% recall the episode in detail.

The HRT Study

The best recent example of the risks of observational research is the experience of the medical community with estrogenic hormone replacement therapy (HRT) in postmenopausal women. All evidence short of RCTs – multiple large prospective cohort studies, many retrospective cohort studies, and the individual clinical experience of the majority of physicians and specialists – agreed that HRT was beneficial in many ways (for osteoporosis, mood, and memory) and not harmful. A large RCT by the Women's Health Initiative (WHI) investigators disproved this belief: the treatment was not effective in any demonstrable way, and it caused harm by increasing the risk of certain cancers. The WHI study also was an observational prospective cohort study, and thus it provided the unique opportunity to compare the best nonrandomized (prospective cohort) and randomized data for the same topic in the same sample. As shown by many previous studies, this comparison showed that observational data (even under the best conditions) inflates efficacy compared to RCTs (Prentice et al. 2006).

Many clinicians are still disturbed by the results of the Women's Health Initiative RCT; some insist that certain subgroups had benefit, which may be the case, although this possibility needs to be interpreted with the caution that is due subgroup analysis (see Chapter 6). But, in the end, this experience is an important cautionary tale about the deep and profound reality of confounding bias, and the limitations of our ability to observe what is really the case in our daily clinical experience.

The Benefits of Observational Research

The case against observational studies should not be overstated, however. Ivory-tower EBM proponents tend to assume that observational studies systematically overestimate effect sizes compared to RCTs in many different conditions and settings. In fact, this kind of generic overestimation has not been empirically shown. One review that assessed the matter came to the opposite conclusion (Benson and Hartz 2000). That analysis looked at 136 studies of 19 treatments in a range of medical specialties (from cardiology to psychiatry); it found that only 2 of the 19 analyses showed inflated effect sizes with observational studies compared to RCTs. In most cases, in fact, RCTs only confirmed what observational studies had already found. Perhaps this consistency may relate more to high-quality observational studies (prospective cohort studies) than to other observational data, but it should be a source of caution for those who would throw away all knowledge except those studies anointed with placebos.

RCTs are the gold standard and the most valid kind of knowledge. But they have their limits. Where they cannot be conducted, observational research, properly understood, is a linchpin of medical knowledge.

The Alchemy of Meta-Analysis

Exercising the right of occasional suppression and slight modification, it is truly absurd to see how plastic a limited number of observations become, in the hands of men with preconceived ideas.

(Sir Francis Galton, 1863; quoted in Stigler 1986, p. 267)

It is an interesting fact that meta-analysis is the product of psychiatry. It was developed specifically to refute a critique, made in the 1960s by the irrepressible psychologist Hans Eysenck, that psychotherapies (mainly psychoanalytic) were ineffective (Hunt 1997). Yet the word "meta-analysis" seems too awe-inspiring for most mental health professionals to even begin to approach it. This need not be the case.

The rationale for meta-analysis is to provide some systematic way of putting together all the scientific literature on a specific topic. Though Eysenck was correct that there are many limitations to meta-analysis, we cannot avoid the fact that we will always be trying to make sense of the scientific literature as a whole, and not just study by study. If we don't use meta-analysis methods, we will inevitably be using some methods to make these judgments, most of which have even more faults than meta-analysis. In the next chapter we will see another totally different mindset, Bayesian statistics, as a way to put all the knowledge base together for clinical practice.

Critics have noted that meta-analysis resembles alchemy (Feinstein 1995): taking the dross of individually negative studies to produce the gold of a positive pooled result. But alchemy led to the science of chemistry and, properly used, meta-analysis can advance our knowledge.

So, let us see what meta-analysis is all about and how it fares compared to other ways of reviewing the scientific literature.

Nonsystematic Reviews

There is likely to be broad consensus that the least acceptable approach to a review of the literature is the classic "selective" review, in which the reviewer selects those articles which agree with his opinion and ignores those which do not. On this approach, any opinion can be supported by selectively choosing among studies in the literature. The opposite of the selective review is the systematic review. In this approach, some effort is made, usually with computerized searching, to identify all studies on a topic. Once all studies are identified (including, ideally, some that may not have been published), then the question is how these studies can be compared.

The simplest approach to reviewing a literature is the "vote count" method: How many studies were positive, and how many negative? The problem with this approach is that it fails to take into account the quality of the various studies (i.e., sample sizes, randomized or not, control of bias, adequacy of statistical testing for chance). The next most rigorous approach is a pooled analysis. This approach corrects for sample size, unlike vote counting, but nothing else. Other features of studies are not assessed, such as bias in design, randomization or not, and so on. Sometimes those features can be controlled by inclusion criteria which might, for instance, limit a pooled analysis to only randomized studies.

Meta-Analysis Defined

Meta-analysis represents an observational study of studies. In other words, one tries to combine the results of many different studies into one summary measure. This is, to some extent, unavoidable in that clinicians and researchers need to try to pull together different studies into some useful summary of the state of the literature on a topic. There are different ways to go about this, with meta-analysis perhaps the most useful, but all reviews also have their limitations.

Apples and Oranges

Meta-analysis weights studies by their samples sizes, but in addition it also corrects for the variability of the data (some studies have smaller standard deviations, and thus their results are more precise and reliable). The problem still remains that studies differ from each other – the problem of "heterogeneity" (sometimes called the "apples and oranges" problem) – which reintroduces confounding bias when the actual results are combined. The main attempts to deal with this problem in meta-analysis are the same as in observational studies. (Randomization is not an option because one cannot randomize studies, only patients within a study.) One option is to exclude certain confounding factors through strict inclusion criteria. For instance, a meta-analysis may only include women, and thus gender is not a confounder; or, perhaps a meta-analysis would be limited to the elderly, thus excluding confounding by younger age. Often, meta-analyses are limited to randomized clinical trials only, as in the Cochrane Collaboration, with the idea being that patient samples will be less heterogeneous in the highly controlled setting of RCTs as opposed to observational studies. Nonetheless, given that meta-analysis itself is an observational study, it is important to realize that the benefits of randomization are lost. Often readers may not realize this point, and thus it may seem that a meta-analysis of 10 RCTs is more meaningful than each RCT alone. However, each large, well-conducted RCT is basically free of confounding bias, while no meta-analysis is completely free of confounding bias. The most meaningful findings are when individual RCTs and the overall meta-analysis all point in the same direction.

Another way to handle the confounding bias of meta-analysis, just as in single observational studies, is to use stratification or regression models, often called meta-regression. For instance, if 10 RCTs exist, but 5 used a crossover design and 5 used a parallel design, one could create a regression model in which the relative risk of benefit with drug versus placebo is obtained corrected for variables of crossover design and parallel design.

Publication Bias

Besides the apples and oranges problem, the other major problem of meta-analysis is the publication bias, or file-drawer, problem. The issue here is that the published literature may not be a valid reflection of the reality of research on a topic because positive studies are published more often than negative studies. This occurs for various reasons. Editors may be more inclined to reject negative studies given the limits of publication space. Researchers may be less inclined to put effort into writing and revising manuscripts of negative studies given the lack of interest engendered by such reports. And, perhaps most importantly, pharmaceutical companies who conduct RCTs have a strong economic motivation *not* to publish negative studies of their drugs. When published, their competitors would likely seize upon negative findings to attack a company's drug, and the cost of preparing and producing such manuscripts would likely be hard to justify to the marketing managers of a for-profit company. In summary, there are many reasons that lead to the systematic suppression of negative treatment studies. Meta-analyses would then be biased toward positive findings for efficacy of treatments. One possible way around this problem that has gradually begun to be implemented in places is to create a data registry where all RCTs conducted on a topic are registered. For studies that are not published, managers of those registries could obtain the actual data from negative studies and store them for the use of systematic reviews and meta-analyses. This possible solution is limited by the fact that it is dependent on the voluntary cooperation of researchers, and in the case the pharmaceutical industry, with a few exceptions, most companies refuse to provide such negative data (Ghaemi et al. 2008a). The patent and privacy laws in the USA protect them on this issue, but this factor makes definitive scientific reviews of evidence difficult to achieve.

Network Meta-analysis: Making It All Even Worse

An especially popular new variation on meta-analysis is "network" meta-analysis. This approach is, in my view, even worse and more invalid than standard meta-analysis. Here's what happens: In standard meta-analysis, if drug x is compared to placebo in 10 different studies, you can pool the results of drug x in those 10 studies and pool the results of placebo in those 10 studies, and add them all up. (Not exactly, because it's not simple addition; but this is the basic concept.) That process, as discussed, has the limitation that each study could be different, with samples that are not the same in various features, such as age or severity of illness or other confounding factors. These differences introduce confounding bias to meta-analysis, called "heterogeneity," which reduces the validity of meta-analysis compared to single randomized trials.

A problem that is common in meta-analysis often is that there aren't enough studies to add up. Instead of 10 studies of drug x versus placebo, there may be only 3 studies. That's not enough to meta-analyze.

Here's where the solution of network meta-analysis comes in, solving this problem but worsening the problem of heterogeneity. Network meta-analysis says "No problem! If there are only three studies of drug x vs placebo, but there are two studies of drug y vs placebo, and four studies of drug z vs placebo, we can just add up the placebo results in all these studies!" So now there are nine studies (three for drug x, two for drug y, and four for drug z) and we can add up all the placebo results in those nine studies. Here's the trick: Now we can compare the three studies of drug x versus *nine studies* of placebo, and two for drug y versus *nine studies* of placebo, and four for drug z versus *nine studies* of placebo. Now even though the drug study results can't be added up, they will have more statistical power because they'll be compared to many more patients in the placebo arm.

Notice that now the network meta-analysis assumes that placebo effects are the same in all different studies, including studies of completely different drugs. This adds another major confounding factor the results, thereby making them even less valid.

Here's a metaphor for how network meta-analysis is likely to be false. Imagine an international soccer tournament, like the Champions League. Suppose Manchester City beats Real Madrid and Real Madrid beats Barcelona; network analysis would then state that Manchester City would beat Barcelona. Of course, in soccer it doesn't work this way; Barcelona could beat Manchester City even though they had lost to Real Madrid (whom Manchester City had beaten).

It doesn't work in soccer, and it doesn't work in nature.

Not only is the claim false because of its false transitive logic, it's false in its claim of relative efficacy. If Manchester City beats Real Madrid 6–0, and Barcelona beats Real Madrid 3–0, then network meta-analysis will conclude that Manchester City will beat Barcelona by 3 goals (6–3 or some other combination of a 3 goal difference).

That's not true in soccer, and that's not true in nature.

Just because drug x is much better than placebo in three studies, and drug z is less better than placebo in four studies, it doesn't mean that drug x is better than drug z. But that's what network meta-analysis will claim.

Network meta-analysis assumes that the placebo effect is the same or similar across studies with different drugs in different samples. This assumption is known to be false.

And that's why network meta-analysis is false.

Clinical example: Network meta-analysis of antidepressants in "major depressive disorder"

Network meta-analysis is now rampant, and many researchers make a living doing it. A classic example was given previously in Chapter 8 on the importance of effect sizes. That review involved *The Lancet* publication on antidepressant efficacy in so-called MDD (Cipriani et al. 2018), which claimed to definitively prove that antidepressants "work" and that it was the best evidence on the subject. In all, 522 RCTs with a larger sample (more than 116,000 participants) and with 21 different antidepressants were examined, with about half of the studies being previously unpublished.

To remind the reader, the study claimed high antidepressant efficacy based on *relative* effect sizes (odds ratios), but in the middle of about 300 pages of the online appendix, the review buried the reality that the absolute effect size (Cohen's d) was small and not clinically meaningful.

Given this general inefficacy found in the study, which the publication ignored, the relative differences between the medications also are not as meaningful as the paper claims, given the analysis just provided of the higher invalidity of network meta-analysis compared to standard meta-analysis. The review found the largest overall absolute benefit with the only tricyclic antidepressant included, amitriptyline, and the lowest overall benefit with reboxetine, a pure noradrenergic antidepressant marketed in Europe and Canada. The study might conclude that amitriptyline is inherently better than reboxetine; maybe, but only if Manchester City could be guaranteed to beat Barcelona, and that they would win by three goals.

Clinical example: Sertraline is the best antidepressant

The same authors previously published another network meta-analysis (Cipriani et al. 2009) which proved – or so it would seem to readers who assumed the validity of network meta-analysis – that some antidepressants clearly are more effective than others; specifically, that escitalopram and sertraline were the most effective antidepressants with the most tolerability, and that fluoxetine and paroxetine had less efficacy, among other agents. The abstract specifically called out sertraline as the best initial choice for depression treatment.

These results were based on a network meta-analysis of 12 drugs with 117 RCTs in almost 26,000 participants. The placebo arms were pooled across all studies as described. Again, the claim is based on the fact that sertraline had a larger effect size of benefit over placebo in its studies than fluoxetine did in its studies, for example. Make sertraline Manchester City, make fluoxetine Barcelona, and make placebo Real Madrid – and you have your claim.

Sertraline is better than fluoxetine only if Manchester City is guaranteed to beat Barcelona, and to win by three goals.

Meta-Analysis As Interpretation

The foregoing example demonstrates the dangers of meta-analysis, as well as some of its benefits. Ultimately, meta-analysis is not the simple quantitative exercise that it may appear to be and that some of its aficionados appear to believe is the case. It involves many, many interpretive judgments – much more than in the usual application of statistical concepts to a single clinical trial. Its real danger, then, as Eysenck tried to emphasize (Eysenck 1994), is that it can put an *end* to discussion, based on biased interpretations cloaked with quantitative authority, rather than leading to more accurate evaluation of available studies. At root, Eysenck points out that what matters is the *quality* of the studies, a matter that is not itself a quantitative question (Eysenck 1994).

Meta-analysis can clarify, and it can be obfuscate. By choosing one's inclusion and exclusion criteria carefully, one can still prove whatever point one wishes. Sometimes meta-analyses of the same topic, published by different researchers, directly conflict with each other. Meta-analysis is a tool, not an answer. We should not let this method control us, doing meta-analyses willy-nilly on any and all topics (as unfortunately appears to be the habit of some researchers), but, rather, cautiously and selectively where the evidence seems amenable to this kind of methodology.

Meta-Analysis Is Less Valid Than RCTs

One last point deserves to be re-emphasized, a point which meta-analysis mavens sometimes dispute, without justification: *Meta-analysis is never more valid than an equally large single RCT*. This is because a single RCT of 500 patients means that the whole sample is randomized and therefore confounding bias should be minimal. But a meta-analysis of 5 different RCTs that add up to a total of 500 patients is *no longer a randomized study*. Meta-analysis is an observational pooling of data; the fact that the data were originally randomized no longer applies once they are pooled. So if they conflict, the results of meta-analysis, despite the fanciness of the word, should never be privileged over a large RCT. In the case of the foregoing example, that methodologically flawed meta-analysis does not come close to the validity of a recently published large RCT of 366 patients randomized to antidepressants versus placebo for bipolar depression, in which, contrary to the meta-analysis, there was no benefit with antidepressants (Sachs et al. 2007).

Statistical Alchemy

Alvan Feinstein (Feinstein 1995) has thoughtfully critiqued meta-analysis in a way that pulls together much of the foregoing discussion. He notes that, after much effort, scientists have come to a consensus about the nature of science; it must have four features: reproducibility, "precise characterization," unbiased comparisons ("internal validity"), and appropriate generalization ("external validity"). Readers will note that he thereby covers the same territory I use in this book as the three organizing principles of statistics: bias, chance, and causation. Meta-analysis, Feinstein argues, ruins all this effort. It does so because it seeks to "convert existing things into something better. 'Significance' can be attained statistically when small group sizes are pooled into big ones; and new scientific hypotheses, that had inconclusive results or that had not been originally tested, can be examined for special subgroups or other entities." These benefits come at the cost, though, of "the removal or destruction of the scientific requirements that have been so carefully developed" (Feinstein 1995, p. 71).

He makes the analogy to alchemy because of "the idea of getting something for nothing, while simultaneously ignoring established scientific principles" (Feinstein 1995, p. 71). He calls this the "free lunch" principle, which makes meta-analysis suspect, along with the "mixed salad" principle, his metaphor for heterogeneity (implying even more drastic differences than apples and oranges).

He notes that meta-analysis violates one of Hill's concepts of causation: the notion of *consistency*. Hill thought that studies should generally find the same result; meta-analysis accepts studies with differing results, and privileges some over others: "With meta-analytic aggregates ... the important inconsistencies are ignored and buried in the statistical agglomeration" (Feinstein 1995, p. 76).

Perhaps most importantly, Feinstein worried that researchers would stop doing better and better studies, and spend all their time trying to wrench truth from meta-analysis of poorly done studies. In effect, meta-analysis is unnecessary where it is valid and unhelpful where it is needed: Where studies are poorly done, meta-analysis is unhelpful, combining only highly heterogeneous and faulty data and thereby producing falsely precise but invalid meta-analytic results. Where studies are well done, meta-analysis is redundant: "My chief complaint ... is that meta-analysis of randomized trials concentrates on a part of the scientific domain that is already reasonably well lit, while ignoring the much larger domain that lies either in darkness or in deceptive glitters" (Feinstein 1995, p. 78).

Feinstein's critique culminates in seeing meta-analysis as a symptom of EBM run amuck, with the Cochrane Collaboration in Oxford as its symbol, a new potential source of Galenic dogmatism, now in statistical guise (Feinstein and Horwitz 1997). When RCTs are simply immediately put into meta-analysis software, and all other studies are ignored, then the only way in which meta-analysis can be legitimate – careful assessment of quality and attention to heterogeneity – is obviated. Quoting the statistician Richard Peto, Feinstein notes that "the painstaking detail of a good meta-analysis 'just isn't possible in the Cochrane collaboration' when the procedures are done 'on an industrial scale'" (Feinstein and Horwitz 1997, p. 534).

Eysenck Again

I had the pleasure of meeting Eysenck, and I will never forget his devotion to statistical research. "You cannot have knowledge," he told me over lunch, "unless you can count it." What about the case report, I asked; is that not knowledge at all? He smiled and held up a single finger: "Even then you can count." Eysenck contributed a lot to empirical research in psychology, personality, and psychiatric genetics. Thus, his reservations about meta-analysis are even more relevant since they do not come from a person averse to statistics, but rather from someone who perhaps knows all too well the limits of statistics.

I will give Eysenck the last word, from a 1994 paper which is among his last writings:

> Rutherford once pointed out that when you needed statistics to make your results significant, you would be better off doing a better experiment. Meta-analyses are often used to recover something from poorly designed studies, studies of insufficient statistical power, studies that give erratic results, and those resulting in apparent contradictions. Occasionally, meta-analysis does give worthwhile results, but all too often it is subject to methodological criticisms. ... Systematic reviews range all the way from highly subjective "traditional" methods to computer-like, completely objective counts of estimates of effect size over all published (and often unpublished) material regardless of quality. Neither extreme seems desirable. There cannot be one best method for fields of study so diverse as those for which meta-analysis has been used. If a medical treatment has an effect so recondite and obscure as to require meta-analysis to establish it, I would not be happy to have it used on me. It would seem better to improve the treatment, and the theory underlying the treatment.
>
> (Eysenck 1994, p. 792)

We can summarize: Meta-analysis can thus be seen as useful in two settings: Where research is ongoing, it can be seen as a stop-gap measure, a temporary summary of the state of the evidence, to be superseded by future larger studies. Where further RCT research is uncommon or unlikely, meta-analysis can serve as a more or less definitive summing up of what we know, and thus it can be used to inform Bayesian methods of decision-making.

Bayesian Statistics: Why Your Opinion Counts

Bayesianism is the dirty little secret of statistics. It is the aunt that no one wants to invite to dinner. If mainstream statistics is akin to democratic socialism, Bayesianism often comes across as something like a Trotskyist fringe group, acknowledged at times but rarely tolerated.

Yet, like so many contrarian views, there are probably important truths in this little-known and less-understood approach to statistics, truths which clinicians in the medical and mental health professions might understand more easily and more objectively than statisticians.

Two Philosophies of Statistics

There are two basic philosophies of statistics: mainstream current statistics views itself as only assessing data and mathematical interpretations of data – this is called *frequentist* statistics; the alternative approach sees data as being interpretable only in terms of other data or other probability judgments – this is *Bayesian* statistics. Most statisticians want science to be based on numbers, not opinions; hence, following Fisher, most mainstream statistical methods are frequentist. This frequentist philosophy is not as pure as statisticians might wish, however; throughout this book, I have emphasized the many points in which traditional statistics – and by this I mean the most hard-nosed, data-driven, frequentist variety – involves subjective judgments, arbitrary cut-offs, and conceptual schema. This happens not just here and there, but frequently and in quite important places (two examples are the p-value cut-off and the null hypothesis definition). But Bayesianism makes subjective judgment part and parcel of the core notion of all statistics: probability. For frequentists, this goes too far. (It might analogize to how capitalists might accept some need for market regulation, but to them socialism seems too extreme.)

In mainstream statistics, the only place where Bayesian concepts are routinely allowed has to do with diagnostic tests (which I will discuss later). More generally, though, there is something special about Bayesian statistics that is worth some effort on the part of clinicians: One might appreciate and even agree with the general wish to base science on hard numbers, not opinions. But clinicians are used to subjectivity and opinions; in fact, much of the instinctive distrust by clinicians of statistics has to do with frequentist assumptions. Bayesian views sit much more comfortably with the unconscious intuitions of clinicians.

Bayes' Theorem

There was once a minister, Reverend Thomas Bayes, who enjoyed mathematics. Living in the mid-eighteenth century, Bayes was interested in the early French notions (e.g., LaPlace) about probability. Bayes discovered something odd: probabilities appeared to be conditional on something else; they did not exist on their own. So if, say, there is a 75% chance that Y will happen, what we are saying is that assuming X, there is a 75% chance that Y will happen. Since X itself is a probability, then we are saying that, assuming (let's say) an 80% chance that X will happen, there is a 75% chance that Y will happen. In Bayes' own words, he defines probability thus: "The probability of any event is the ratio between the value at which an expectation depending on the happening of the event ought to be computed, and the value of the thing expected upon its happening" (Barnard and Bayes 1958, p. 293). The derivation of the mathematical formula – called Bayes' theorem – will not concern us here; suffice it to say that as a matter of mathematics, Bayes' concept is thought to be sound. Stated conceptually, his theorem is that given a prior probability X, the observation of event Y produces a posterior probability Z.

This might be simplified, following Salsburg (2001a, p. 134), as follows:
"Prior probability →Data →Posterior probability"

Salsburg emphasizes how Bayes' theorem reflects how most humans actually think: "The Bayesian approach is to start with a prior set of probabilities in the mind of a given person. Next, that person observes or experiments and produces data. The data are then used to modify the prior probabilities, producing a posterior set of probabilities" (Salsburg 2001a, p. 134).

Normally statistics only have to do with Y and Z. We observe certain events Y, and we then infer the probability of that event, or the probability of that event occurring by chance, or some other probability (Z) related to that event. What Bayes adds is an initial probability of the event, a *prior probability*, before we even observe anything. How can this be? And what is this prior probability?

Bayes himself apparently was not sure what to make of the results of his mathematical work. He never published his material and apparently rarely spoke of it. It came to light after his death and in the nineteenth century had a good deal of influence in the newly developing field of statistics. In the early twentieth century, as the modern foundations of statistics began to be laid by Karl Pearson and Ronald Fisher, however, their first target, and one which they viewed with great animus, was Thomas Bayes.

The Attack on Bayes

Bayes' theorem was seen by Pearson and Fisher as dangerous because it introduced *subjectivity* into statistics, and not here and there, or peripherally, but centrally, into the very basic concept that underlies all statistics: probability. The prior probability seems suspiciously like simply one's opinion before observing the data. Pearson and Fisher could agree that if we want statistics to form the basis of modern science, especially in clinical medicine, then we want to base statistics on data and on defensible mathematical formulae that interpret the data, but *not* on simply one's opinion.

The concern has to do with how we establish prior probability: what is it based on? The most obvious answer is that it involves "personal probability." The extreme view, developed by the statistician L. J. Savage is that "there are no such things as proven scientific facts ....There are only statements, about which people who call themselves scientists associate a high probability" (Salsburg 2001a, p. 133). This is one extreme of Bayesian probability, the most *subjectivist* variety. We might term the other extreme *objectivist*, for it minimizes the subjective opinion of any individual; developed by John Maynard Keynes, the famous economist, this kind of Bayesian probability appeals to me.

Keynes' view was that personal probability should not be the view that any person happens to hold, but rather "the degree of belief that an educated person in a given culture can be expected to hold" (Salsburg 2001a, pp. 133–4). This is similar to Charles Sanders Peirce's view that the truth is what the consensus of community of investigators believes to be the case at the limit of scientific investigation. Peirce, like Keynes, was arguing that for scientific concepts in physics, for instance, the opinion of the construction worker does not count the same as the opinion of a professor of physics. What matters is the consensus of those who are of a similar background and have a similar knowledge base and are engaged in similar efforts to know.

I would take Keynes and Peirce one step further, so as to place Bayesian statistics on even more objective ground, and thus to emphasize to readers that it is valid and, in many ways, not in conflict with standard frequentist statistics. The middle and final terms of Bayes' theorem, as mentioned, are accepted by frequentist mainstream statistics. Data are numbers, not opinions, and certain probabilities can be inferred based on the data. The issue is the prior probability. What if we assert that the prior probability is also solely based on the results of frequentist statistics – that is, that it is based on the state of the scientific literature? We might use meta-analysis of all available RCTs, for instance, as our prior probability on a given topic. Then a new study would lead to a posterior probability after we incorporate those results with the prior status quo as described in a previous meta-analysis. In that way, the Bayesian structure is used, but with nonsubjective and frequentist content. Of course, there will always be some subjectivity to any interpretation, such as meta-analysis, but that level of subjectivity is irremovable and inherent in any kind of statistics, including frequentist methods.

Readers may choose whichever approach they prefer, but I think a case can at least be made for using Bayesian methods with prior probabilities based on the state of the objective scientific literature, and, in doing so, we would not be violating the standards of frequentist mainstream statistics.

Bayesianism in Psychiatric Practice

Let us pause. Before we reject personal probability as too opinioned, or think of Bayesian approaches as unnecessary or too complex, let me point out that most clinicians – doctors and mental health professionals – operate this way. And accepting personal probability is not equivalent to saying that we must accept a complete relativism about what is probable. Here is an example from a supervision session I recently conducted with a psychiatry resident, Jane, who described a patient of long standing in our outpatient psychiatry clinic: "No one knows what to do with him," she began. "You won't either, because no one knows the true diagnosis." He was a poor historian and had no family available for corroboration, so important past details of his history could not be obtained. Yet, as she described his history, a few salient points became clear: he had failed to respond to numerous antidepressants for repeated major depressive episodes, which had led to 6 hospitalizations, beginning at age 22. He had taken all antidepressants, all antipsychotics, and all mood stabilizers. He did not have chronic psychotic symptoms, though possibly had brief such symptoms during his hospitalizations. He had encephalitis at age 17. His family history was unknown. He probably had become manic on an antidepressant once, with marked overactivity and hypersexuality just after taking it, compared to no such behavior before or since.

We could only know those facts with reasonable probability. So, beginning with the differential diagnosis of recurrent severe depression, I asked her what the possibilities were; it soon became clear that unipolar depression ("major depressive disorder") was the prime diagnosis. When asked about the alternatives, she acknowledged the need to rule out bipolar disorder and secondary mood disorder (depression due to medical illness). Her supposition had been that he had failed to respond to antidepressants for his unipolar depression due to likely concomitant personality disorder, though the nature of that condition was unclear (he did not have classic features of borderline or antisocial personality disorder). Though I acknowledged that possibility, I asked her to think back to the mood disorder differential first.

Let's begin with the conditions that need to be ruled out, I said. The only possible medical illness that could be relevant was encephalitis. Is encephalitis associated with recurrent severe major depressive episodes more than two decades later, I asked? We both acknowledged that this was improbable on the basis of the known scientific evidence. So, if we begin with initial complete uncertainty about the role of encephalitis in this recurrent depressive illness, we might start at the 50–50 mark of probability. After consulting the known scientific literature, we then conclude that encephalitis is lower than 50% in probability; if we had to quantify our own personal probability, perhaps it would fall to 20% or less given the absence of any evidence suggesting an encephalitis/long-term recurrent severe depressive illness connection. This is a Bayesian judgment and can be depicted visually, with 0% reflecting no likelihood of the diagnosis and 100% reflecting absolute certainty of the diagnosis (see Figure 13.1).

Next, one could turn to the bipolar disorder differential diagnosis. If we began again with a neutral attitude of complete uncertainty, our anterior probability would be at the 50–50 mark. Beginning to look at the highly probable facts of the clinical history, two facts stand out: antidepressant-induced mania and nonresponse to multiple therapeutic trials of antidepressants (documented in the outpatient records). We can then turn again to known scientific knowledge: antidepressant-induced mania occurs in <1% of persons with unipolar depression, but in 5–50% of persons with bipolar disorder. Thus, it is 5–50-fold more likely that bipolar disorder is the diagnosis rather than unipolar depression based on that fact. Treatment nonresponse to 3 or more adequate antidepressant trials are associated, in some studies, with a 25–50% likelihood of misdiagnosed bipolar disorder, the most common feature associated with such treatment resistance. Thus, both clinical features would make the probability of bipolar disorder higher, not lower. So we would move from the 50% mark closer to the 100% mark. Depending on the strength of the scientific literature, the quality of the studies, the amount of replication, and our own interpretation of that literature, we might move more or less toward 100%, but the direction of movement can only go one way, toward increased probability of diagnosis. If I had to quantify for myself, I might visually depict it as shown in Figure 13.2.

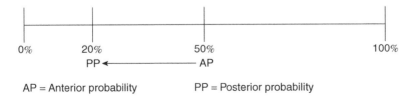

AP = Anterior probability   PP = Posterior probability

Figure 13.1 Probability of diagnosis of encephalitis-induced mood disorder

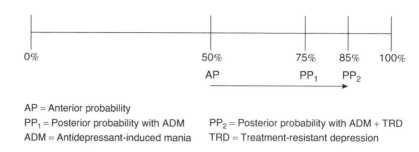

AP = Anterior probability
PP₁ = Posterior probability with ADM   PP₂ = Posterior probability with ADM + TRD
ADM = Antidepressant-induced mania   TRD = Treatment-resistant depression

Figure 13.2 Probability of diagnosis of bipolar disorder

In my personal probability, the likelihood of bipolar disorder increases to the point where it is highly likely. If we assume that at 80% or above likelihood we might make major treatment changes, I might then make major changes in this person's treatment and insist upon them due to my confidence based on this high level of probability. Now, it might be objected that the threshold at which we might change treatments is again subjective, a matter of personal probability, but it is not completely arbitrary: 95% certainty means more than 65% certainty. We can likely agree on a conceptually sound level of certainty, perhaps 80% and above, much as we do in frequentist statistics for concepts such as power or statistical significance.

Once I spelled out this Bayesian rationale for diagnostic probability, Jane was convinced, somewhat against her will. Why had she not reached the same conclusions earlier, and why was she still resistant? Mainly, I believe, it had to do with the sloppy intuitive approach to diagnosis which is so common in clinical practice, combined with the harmful impact of her own assumed biases. In addition, Jane did not know about the studies conducted on antidepressant-induced mania and treatment-resistant depression. So there was a problem with lack of factual knowledge, which is usually what methods like evidence-based medicine (EBM) seek to emphasize, but, perhaps more importantly, there was also a conceptual problem with unexamined biases. The Bayesian approach brings out these unexamined biases and thus minimizes them. If we were to depict Jane's Bayesian diagnostic process before we had discussed the case, it would have been something along the lines in Figure 13.3. We start with a low probability of bipolar disorder because she was biased against the diagnosis (in general, it seems; but also most clearly in relation to this patient, for whom she intuitively preferred a personality disorder diagnosis). She started out with a very low probability, did not know that treatment-resistant depression (TRD) would increase it, and felt that antidepressant-induced mania (ADM) would increase it only slightly. Thus, her Bayesian process as regards bipolar disorder might be depictable as in Figure 13.3.

This is her personal probability but, based on the known scientific literature, one cannot plausibly argue that her personal probability was as valid as mine.

Now some readers might say, "Wait: You say that she was biased against the bipolar diagnosis, which led her Bayesian reasoning to fail to reach probable levels even with the history of ADM and TRD. Are not you biased in favor of the bipolar diagnosis? Could not that be why your probabilities ended up closer to 100%?" This would be the case if my anterior initial probability was above 50%. If I had started at 80% probability, then the ADM and TRD features of this patient's illness might take me to 99% as a posterior probability;

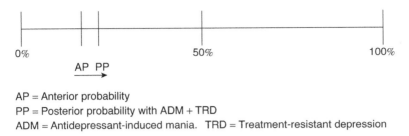

AP = Anterior probability
PP = Posterior probability with ADM + TRD
ADM = Antidepressant-induced mania. TRD = Treatment-resistant depression

Figure 13.3 Jane's probability of diagnosis of bipolar disorder

indeed, that might be the case if there was initial bias. But I started at the 50–50 probability level, not higher. This is the neutral point, at which no bias toward any diagnosis is the case. Recall that I also started at 50–50 when assessing the likelihood of encephalitis-induced mood disorder.

If we were to repeat the same Bayesian diagrams with the possible diagnosis of unipolar depression ("major depressive disorder"), we could also begin at the 50–50 level, but we would quickly move, based on the frequentist scientific literature, to a lower probability level due to TRD and ADM.

The main point of this discussion is that the use of Bayesian statistics in this way is not an exercise in completely arbitrary subjectivity. In fact, it decreases our arbitrary, subjective, intuitive approach to clinical practice by forcing us to be explicit about our assumptions and to make at least probabilistic quantifications about them. Further, it relies on the scientific literature, which is based on frequentist methods; it utilizes nonsubjective knowledge to inform its subjective probabilistic conclusions (Goodman 1999).

The Ping-Pong Effect

The two approaches – classical and Bayesian – are based on different conceptual assumptions about the nature of statistical interpretation. Neither approach is definitively right or wrong. In fact, the Bayesian approach not only highlights the limitations of the frequentist approach, it also shows why classical frequentist statistics is limited: Examples of these mainstream statistical blindspots, the author continues, are subgroup analyses and multiple comparisons (discussed in Chapter 8). Most statisticians, being frequentists, err on the side of the null hypothesis: unless they are more than 95% certain, they do not consider a finding as notable. This is like, on the visual depictions of diagnostic decision-making given earlier, always starting at the 5% mark – that is, always having a low prior probability that something is the case. Then if positive data are produced, one would jump to the opposite end and be at the 95% mark, with a very high posterior probability that something is the case. Then again, if the next study is negative, one would jump back to the 5% mark. This ping-pong effect underlies the confusion of many clinicians about opposing results of different scientific studies, as depicted in Figure 13.4. If they began in the middle of the visual axis of certainty, however, clinicians would be less liable to be confused, because conflicting data would cancel out and clinicians would throughout remain in the stable state of uncertainty around the 50–50 mark.

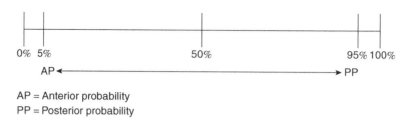

AP = Anterior probability
PP = Posterior probability

Figure 13.4 The ping-pong effect: Frequentist interpretation of conflicting studies

Diagnostic Tests

Now I will apply Bayesian methods statistically where they are most clear-cut, in assessing diagnostic screening tests, with my example being patient self-report questionnaires designed to detect bipolar disorder (the Mood Disorders Questionnaire [MDQ], and the Bipolar Spectrum Diagnostic Scale [BSDS]). In a study, my colleague Jim Phelps and I applied Bayesian statistical concepts to assess how such a screening tool might be appropriately used; in the process, we also saw how classical frequentist statistical assumptions led clinicians and researchers to make grave errors of interpretation (Phelps and Ghaemi 2006).

Usually those screening tools were reported in terms of the classic frequentist statistics of sensitivity (if the patient has the disease, is the test positive?) and specificity (if the patient does not have the disease, is the test negative?). With high scores on both counts, researchers and clinicians often concluded that positive scores, without any further clinical evaluation, indicated presence of bipolar disorder. Such research was even published in very high-profile scientific journals (Das et al. 2005).

Predictive value, on the other hand, is a Bayesian concept: if the test is positive, how frequently do patients have the disease? (And, if negative, how frequently do they not have it?) It turns out that the answer varies depending on the circumstances, as is the case with Bayesian statistics, unlike classical frequentist statistics: The number does not exist in a vacuum.

Figure 13.5 presents predictive values relative to prevalence, using the sensitivity and specificity data from each of the four studies.

As follows from Bayesian principles, predictive values are inversely affected by prevalence: negative predictive values (NPVs) are low and positive predictive values (PPVs) are high at low prevalence; whereas PPVs are high and NPVs are low at high prevalence. However, PPV is much more sensitive to prevalence than NPV, as manifest in the slope of the respective curves. At low prevalence, which is most relevant to the primary care medicine setting, the sensitivity and specificity of the test has little impact on negative predictive value: all the reported data yield predictive values between 0.92 and 0.97. Similarly, at low prevalence, positive predictive value is low regardless of the sensitivity and specificity data used.

The analysis presented here demonstrates that the MDQ and BSDS perform well at low prevalence (as in the primary care setting), where their strong negative predictive values can effectively screen out bipolar disorder. When given to a patient who arouses little clinical suspicion of bipolar disorder, a negative MDQ will generally help accomplish just what the FDA has recommended prior to administration of antidepressants: the likelihood of bipolar disorder is low, but will likely be made lower still by the administration of the test.

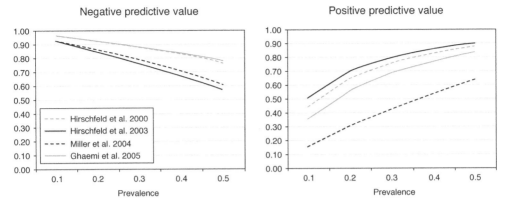

Figure 13.5 Negative versus positive predictive value. From Phelps and Ghaemi (2006) with permission Elsevier. Copyright 2006.

However, a weakness of these tests is also obvious: a positive result, when the clinician is not very suspicious that bipolar disorder is present, has a very high likelihood of being a false positive. This is so regardless of which sensitivity and specificity data one chooses to use. Yet this is a very likely scenario in primary care if the test is used broadly, for example in patients who do not present with depression, or in the bipolar screening the FDA has advocated. Therefore, any presentation of the MDQ or BSDS as tools for bipolar screening should be accompanied by a reminder that positive results are not bipolar diagnoses – a point that is sometimes not prominent in pharmaceutical marketing of the MDQ. One available version of the MDQ makes this point to the patient even before the provider scores it.

In sum, the performance of screening instruments such as the MDQ and BSDS depend not only on their sensitivity and specificity, which are properties of the tests themselves, but also on the prevalence of the illness for which one is screening, as predicted by Bayesian principles.

Honing Our Prior Probabilities

I have applied this approach to the problem of difficult diagnoses, such as bipolar disorder in psychiatry. Because prior clinical probability is so important in the process of diagnosing bipolar disorder, it is even more important to acknowledge that clinicians appear to be inadequately trained or proficient in recognizing bipolar disorder. Much more clinical research exists to suggest that bipolar disorder is underdiagnosed rather than overdiagnosed. The underdiagnosis rate has been confirmed to be about 40% in various studies, with about a decade elapsing from the first visit to a mental health professional after an initial manic episode, and the appropriate diagnosis of bipolar disorder. Part of this underdiagnosis likely relates to patients' lack of insight, whereby they deny or fail to describe manic symptoms. Data exist showing that family members report manic symptoms twice as frequently as patients, and thus family report is essential in the diagnostic assessment of bipolar disorder. But in part this is also due to a lack of systematic assessment of hypomanic and manic symptoms on the part of clinicians, in favor of a simpler but fallible "prototype" or "pattern recognition" approach to diagnosis ("she does not look bipolar") (Sprock 1988).

Another common clinical approach which limits diagnostic accuracy is to focus solely on signs or symptoms of mania in assessing the potential diagnosis of bipolar disorder. It is just as important to assess other important diagnostic validators associated with bipolar disorder: family history of bipolar disorder, course of illness (early age of onset, highly recurrent and brief depressive episodes, psychotic depression, postpartum onset), and antidepressant treatment response (especially mania, tolerance, and nonresponse). All of these factors should be considered as a clinician develops their "hunch" about the likelihood of bipolarity in a patient. If screening tools are used in lieu of this process, their accuracy will be limited.

It appears from this analysis that a clinician's prior probability estimate (based on clinical history, baseline clinical information, past treatment response, or other clinical impressions) about the likelihood of bipolar disorder in a particular patient has as much impact on the clinical performance of the MDQ or BSDS as the test's sensitivity and specificity (and in most cases, more). In practice, clinicians are Bayesians (often without realizing it). If their prior probabilities are low, then these scales more effectively rule out than rule in bipolar disorder. If their prior probabilities are moderate, then these scales may help identify true positive cases. If their prior probabilities are high, then these scales are less relevant. Any improvement in clinicians' ability to form an accurate clinical impression will improve the performance of these tests. Therefore, one way to address concerns about the psychometric properties of these screening tests is to help psychiatrists and primary care providers with finding, understanding, and interpreting clinical clues of bipolar disorder.

Bayesian Decision-Making

John Maynard Keynes is famous as an economist; he arguably saved the world in the Great Depression as he articulated ways that government could ameliorate the capitalist market. Yet, beyond economics, Keynes wrote a major work on probability, and essentially worked out an objectivist approach to Bayesian statistics. Some of his insights in economics may be due to the power of this statistical method.

Clinical medicine would benefit from paying attention to the power of Bayesian statistics. Our current ignorance of it would be as if economists only read Adam Smith and obsessed about the self-regulating aspects of the free market, never entertaining any Keynesian notions about the limitations of the unregulated free market. Bayesian statistics can lead us where frequentist statistics has led us aground. And, perhaps best of all, we clinicians may be more attuned to Bayesian styles of thinking than most statisticians, and thus we can incorporate it more easily.

Put another way, Bayesian statistics provide a way of translating scientific research into practical thinking. For a clinician, a p-value of 0.04 versus 0.12 tells him very little about how that study should impact his decision-making. Indeed, one of the problems with applying statistics to clinical medicine is that the quantitative power of statistical calculations is often clinically irrelevant. If I say the p-value is 0.038957629376, this highly precise number is no more relevant than p = 0.04. Perhaps even more importantly, clinicians, and human beings in general, cannot make probability discriminations on the order of 5% or 10% or so. We might have the data to make such claims, but the brain of the working clinician cannot "see" such data; the clinician cannot discriminate such data in the real world.

This reality is captured in the large psychological literature on decision-making. Much of this research has to do with concepts such as "heuristics": studies of how people actually make decisions and of how probabilities are actually understood by real people (like doctors and clinicians) in the real world. One conclusion from this extensive psychological and statistical research on how humans understand probability is that we human beings are able to distinguish only five basic concepts in probability:

> Surely true
> More probable than not
> As probable as not
> Less probable than not
> Surely false.
>
> *(Salsburg 2001a, p. 307)*

Bayesian thinking is a way to get us into these mindsets, to acknowledge how we think, and to help us arrive, as validly as possible, at one of these probability assessments in our clinical practice. Frequentist statistics may want to be more precise, to say that there is a 10% probability of Y and a 25% probability of Z. But our brains cannot make out that difference. If this is correct, then "many of the techniques of statistical analysis that are standard practice are useless, since they only serve to produce distinctions below the level of human perception" (Salsburg 2001a, p. 307).

Ultimately, a clinician who wants to understand statistics, and to use it in clinical practice, is well-prepared to use Bayesian methods. Bayesian thinking straddles the gulf between the excessive adoration of numbers viewed as truth, so frequent in the world of statistics, and the arbitrary intuitive approach to decision-making for individual patients, the long-held province of the clinician. Instead, Bayesian methods allow clinicians to be more quantitatively sound, and they force statisticians to realize that numbers are not enough. A Bayesian approach *is* what happens in the work of a statistically informed clinician.

The Bayesian Id

We clinicians are all Bayesians, whether we realize it or not, much as Freud showed that we humans all have unconscious emotions. The statistician Jacob Cohen implied this analogy with his term "the Bayesian Id" (Cohen 1994).

Here, readers have mulled over the limitations of hypothesis-testing approaches in medical statistics, they have learned about different philosophies of science as they apply to statistics, and they now know what Bayesian statistics mean. After these three steps, readers can perhaps appreciate what Cohen meant when he said that modern statistics has a "hybrid logic," "a mishmash of Fisher and Neyman-Pearson, with invalid Bayesian interpretation" (Cohen 1994, p. 998). Let me spell this out.

Recall that Fisher invented p-values, and Neyman and Pearson devised the null hypothesis (NH) method to show how p-values could be used. The two approaches do not necessarily flow: Fisher felt null hypotheses were a conceptual excrescence, and that p-values could stand alone, as long as they were applied in RCTs. We might add that Hill showed, in the debate with Fisher over cigarettes, that RCTs were not sufficient, or even necessary, to prove causation. Modern statistics assumes that p-values and hypothesis-testing is legitimate, however, but what did Cohen mean about the Bayesian id?

Perhaps he meant that although we practice the frequentist philosophy of p-values and null hypothesis methods, we always, against our will, apply the unconscious Bayesian method of judging the results based on our personal biases. Recall that when we conduct standard frequentist statistics, we ask the following question: Assuming the null hypothesis is true, how likely is it that we would have observed these data? But we tend to interpret the results in reverse: Given these observed data, how likely is it that the NH is true? We know we are not supposed to do this, we are told not to do this – but our statistical id keeps doing it. Cohen makes this point: "When one rejects [the NH], one wants to conclude that [the NH] is unlikely, say, $p < 0.01$. The very reason the statistical test is done is to be able to reject [the NH] because of its unlikelihood!" (Cohen 1994, p. 998). But here we have become Bayesian: we do a study, observe some results, and then try to infer some probability that the NH is false. We are inferring a probability *based on* the data (Bayesian statistics); we are not inferring the probability *of* the data (frequentist statistics): "But that is the posterior probability, available only through Bayes' theorem, for which one needs to know the probability of the null hypothesis before the experiment, the 'prior' probability" (Cohen 1994, p. 998).

What is the probability of the NH before we do our study? That is a question never asked by Neyman and Pearson and decades of their disciples in hypothesis-testing statistics. The orthodox answer is: 100%; because we have to *assume* that the NH is correct. But, given that we do research to find new facts, to reject the NH, the reality is that we do not believe that the probability of the NH is 100%. If so, we are forced to engage in Bayesian reasoning, and we have to provide some prior estimate for the NH *before* we observe the data.

What could that prior estimate be, without dropping us into the mire of everyone's subjective opinions? As described earlier in this chapter, it could be the consensus of previous empirical studies, or the population prevalence of a diagnosis. Whatever it is, we are better off acknowledging the existence of our Bayesian id and trying to make it conscious, rather than continuing to live in the dream world of hypothesis-testing statistics.

The unexamined qualitative intuitions that spring from our personal biases are dangerous things. Frequentist statistics wants to imagine that those subjective parts of research and practice do not exist; Bayesian statistics acknowledges them, and shows us how we can minimize the harm they produce and maximally utilize the availability of objective scientific evidence.

Reverend Bayes buried his theorem. Perhaps we should bring it back to life.

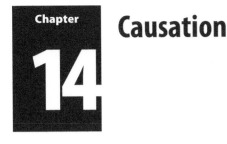

Causation

The whole point of all of the foregoing – of all of the ins and outs of RCTs, and the rigors of regression – is to produce results that allow us to say that something causes something else. All of statistics until this point is about allowing us to infer causation, to make us feel ready to do so. But those efforts – RCTs and regression and the like – do not automatically allow us to infer causation. Causation itself is a separate matter, one which we need to consider – a third hurdle (after bias and chance) which we must overcome before we can say we are finished.

Hume's Fallacy

Causation is essentially a philosophical, not a statistical, problem. Here we see again a key spot where statistics itself does not provide the answers, but we must go outside statistics in order to understand statistics.

The concept of causation may initially seem simple. My daughter, looking over my shoulder at this chapter title, asked "What does causation mean? Well, it means that something caused something. Right?" "Well, yes," I replied. "That's simple, then," she said. "Even an eight-year-old can figure that out."

It seems simple. If I throw a brick at a window, the window breaks: the brick *caused* the window to break. The sun rises every morning and night is replaced by day. The sun *causes* daylight. The word comes from the Latin *causa*, which throws little light on its meaning, except perhaps that it also means "reason." A cause is a reason, but, as we also know by common sense, there are many reasons for many things. There is not just one reason in every case that causes something to happen. The first common-sense intuition we must then recognize is that causation can mean *a* cause and it can mean *many* causes. It does not necessarily mean *the* cause (Doll 2002).

The instincts of common sense were dethroned in the eighteenth century by the philosopher David Hume, who noted that our intuitions about one thing causing another involved an empirical "constant conjunction" of the two events, but no inherent metaphysical link between the two. Every day, the sun rises. A day passes, the sun rises again. There is a constant conjunction, but this in no way proves that some day the sun might not rise: We can call this *Hume's fallacy*.

In other words, observations in the real world cannot prove that one thing causes another; *induction* fails. Hume's critique led many philosophers to search for *deduction* of causality, as in mathematical proofs. Yet the force of his arguments for activities in the world of time and space, such as science, have not lessened with time, and they are central to understanding the uses and limits of statistics in medicine and psychiatry. (I will give more attention to this matter in the next chapter.)

The Tobacco Wars

These two facts – the recognition that induction can be faulty, and the mistaken assumption that causation has to imply *the* cause – have led to much unnecessary scientific conflict over the years. Even Ronald Fisher, the brilliant founder of modern statistics, did not fathom it. In his later life (the 1950s and 1960s), Fisher became a loud critic of those who used his methods to suggest a link between cigarette smoking and lung cancer. Of course, there is no one-to-one connection. Many smokers never develop lung cancer, and some people who have never smoked develop lung cancer. These facts led Fisher to doubt the claimed association. Cigarette smoking did not *cause* lung cancer, Fisher argued, because he thought it had to be *the* cause, the one and only cause, with no other causes. As noted previously (Chapter 7), part of Fisher's scientific concern also was that he felt that the concept of *statistical significance* (p-values) could only be applied in the setting of a randomized clinical trial (RCT). Its application in a completely observational setting, as with cigarette smoking, seemed to him inappropriate. Fisher's view was partly limited by the fact that he did not appreciate the rise of a new discipline, related to but different from statistics: the field of clinical epidemiology. Its founder, A. Bradford Hill, was on the other side of this debate of giants. The conflict over cigarette smoking led Hill to later formulate a list of factors that help us in understanding causation.

We can now, with the advantage of hindsight, look back on this debate and use it to inform how we understand current debates. Today, almost everyone accepts that cigarette smoking causes lung cancer; it is not the *only* cause (other environmental toxins can do so too, and in rare cases purely genetic causation occurs), but it is the *main* cause. In 1950, the first strong piece of evidence to support the link was a case-control study conducted in London. In that study, Hill and his colleague Richard Doll examined 20 London hospitals, identified 709 patients with lung cancer, and matched them by age and gender to 709 patients without lung cancer. They found an association between how many cigarettes had been reported to be smoked and lung cancer. It was not definitive, it was not a 100% connection, but it was present far beyond what could be expected by chance. The key issue was bias. The term "confounding bias" had not been invented yet, but the concept was out there: Could there be other causes of the apparent relationship?

Statistics Versus Epidemiology

Hill and Doll argued that other causes that could completely, or almost completely, explain that their findings were implausible. But there were many weaknesses in their claim. Firstly, no animal studies had identified specific carcinogens in cigarette smoke. Second, the tobacco industry argued that their main source of data was patient recall about past smoking habits: patient recall is known to be faulty. Third, again said the industry, other plausible causes existed, such as environmental pollution, which had increased in the same time frame, and which correlated with the finding that lung cancer was present more in cities than in rural areas. Fisher finally weighed in by adding the other possibility of genetic susceptibility, which he had identified as present in twin studies.

Hill and Doll faced a problem: How can you prove causation in clinical epidemiology? Put another way, how can you prove that anything causes anything else when you are dealing with human beings? With animals, one could control for genetics by breeding for specific genetic types; one can control the environment in a laboratory as well, so that animals can be studied such that they only differ on one feature (the experimental question).

But such experiments are neither feasible nor ethical with humans. How can we ever prove that something causes a disease in humans?

This is the problem of clinical epidemiology. And the conflict between Fisher and Hill shows that statistics are not enough. The numbers can never give the complete answer, *because they are never definitive*. Robert Frost got it right. Statistics, by nature, are never absolute: they are about measuring the probability of error; they can never remove error.

Thus, if one wants to be certain, or very very certain, as in a case where human liberties are being restricted (your rights to cigarette smoking are curtailed, for instance), we seem to have a problem. Fisher, seeing the statistical limits of certainty, felt that it would be hard to prove causation in medical disease. Hill, knowing those same limits, set out to devise a solution.

We have here also, by the way, the source of the philosophical conflict between the two fields of statistics and clinical epidemiology. This is often not obvious to doctors or clinicians, but it is relevant to them. For, with many research questions, if clinicians ask a statistician they will get a different answer than if they ask an epidemiologist; this can especially be the case when one is concerned with interpreting a number of different studies, as in the Fisher vs Hill debate. One solution is to recognize a division of labor: Statisticians are best trained in analyzing the results of a study and in focusing on the risks of chance; epidemiologists are best trained in designing studies and in focusing on the risks of bias. Or, put another way, statisticians are most trained in the conduct of randomized clinical trials and tend to think with hypothesis testing methods; epidemiologists are most trained in the conduct of observational cohort studies and tend to think with descriptive effect estimation methods. The two groups are the Red Sox and Yankees of medical research, and clinicians need to be willing to speak with and understand the perspectives of both of them.

Hill's Concepts of Causation

Now let's turn to what Hill had to say about causation, beginning with a few words about the man. A. Bradford Hill is generally seen as the founder of modern medical epidemiology; modern medicine would be inconceivable without him, and so too would medical statistics. If Fisher invented the ideas, such as randomization, Hill applied them to clinical medicine and worked out their meaning in that context. (One might say that Hill played Lenin to Fisher's Marx.) A single achievement of his would have sufficed to mark the successful career of another man, but Hill was truly revolutionary in his impact. He brought randomization to clinical medical research, conducting the first RCT in 1948 on streptomycin for pneumonia. This, in itself, is like the French Revolution for modern medicine. Yet, in addition to showing how RCTs can bring us closer to the truth – in a way, founding medical statistics in the process – he also realized that much of medicine was not amenable to RCTs, and thus he showed us how to apply statistical methods effectively in observational settings – thus founding clinical epidemiology in the process. This would be the second great revolution of modern medicine. And, in the process, by demonstrating the link between cigarette smoking and lung cancer, Hill rooted out the most deadly preventable illness of the modern era.

With that background, we can listen to what he had to say about the evidence needed to conclude that causation is present in clinical research.

It is a commonplace in statistics that association does not necessarily imply causation. The question, then, is: When does it? This was the topic of a presidential address Hill gave to the Royal Society of Medicine in London: "The Environment and Disease: Association or Causation?" (Hill 1965). Hill first abjures "a philosophical discussion of the meaning of 'causation,'" which we leave for the next chapter. He then defines the practical question for physicians as "whether the frequency of the undesirable event B will be influenced by a change in the environmental feature A" (Hill 1965, p. 295). If we observe an association through observation, unlikely to have occurred by chance, the question is how can we then claim causation? Hill enumerates the ingredients of causation:

1. *Strength of the association*: Smoking increases the likelihood of lung cancer about 10-fold, while it increased the likelihood of heart attack about 2-fold. A very large effect, such as 10-fold or higher, should be seen as strong evidence of causation, Hill argues, unless one can identify some other feature (a confounding factor) directly associated with the proposed cause. With such a large effect size, such confounding factors should be relatively easy to detect, says Hill, thus allowing us "to reject the vague contention of the armchair critic 'you can't prove it, there *may* be such a feature'" Hill 1965, p. 296). (Surely he was thinking of Ronald Fisher here.)

   The reverse does not hold: "We must not be too ready to dismiss a cause-and-effect hypothesis merely on the grounds that the observed association appears to be slight. There are many occasions in medicine when this is in truth so. Relatively few persons harbouring the meningococcus fall sick of meningococcal meningitis" (Hill 1965, p. 296). A strong association makes causation likely; a weak association does not, by itself, make causation unlikely.

2. *Consistency of the association*: This reflects replication – "Has it been repeatedly observed by different persons, in different places, circumstances and times?" (Hill 1965, p. 296). The key to replication, though, is not to replicate using *the exact same* methods, but rather to replicate using *different* methods. Thus, for instance, biased studies are easily replicated; bias reflects *systematic* error, so repetition of a biased study will *systematically* produce the same error. Thus, one nonrandomized observational study found that antidepressant discontinuation in bipolar depression led to depressive recurrence (Altshuler et al. 2003). Another nonrandomized observational study "replicated" the same finding (Joffe et al. 2005). The researchers mistakenly viewed this as strengthening inference of causation. What would strengthen the observational finding would be if randomized data found the same result (which did not occur; Ghaemi et al. 2008). In the case of RCTs, replication by other RCTs would count as improving strength of causation, but again preferably with some differences, such as different dosages or somewhat different patient populations. Again, since no feature is an essential feature of causation, replication is not a *sine qua non*: "there will be occasions when repetition is absent or impossible and yet we should not hesitate to draw conclusions" (Hill 1965, p. 297). This occurs with rare events: if lamotrigine causes Stevens-Johnson syndrome in about 1 in 1,000 persons, statistically significant replication would require a study in which the drug is given to about 3,200 persons, assuming a small standard deviation. This kind of replication is not only unethical, but impossible – another example of the limitations of the p-value approach to statistics, another reason to realize that the concept of "statistical significance" is very limited in its meaning. Causation is a much more important, and inclusive, concept.

3. *Specificity of the association*: Smoking causes lung cancer, not hives. However, this factor should not be over-emphasized because some exposures can cause many

effects: smoking turns out to increase the risk of a range of cancers, not just limited to the lungs. Again, a positive finding rules in causation much more strongly than a negative finding would rule it out: "if specificity exists we may be able to draw conclusions without hesitation; if it is not apparent, we are not thereby necessarily left sitting irresolutely on the fence" (Hill 1965, p. 297).

4. *Temporality*: In the world of time and space, causes precede effects, so unidirectionality in time is important. Fisher once argued that the association between lung cancer and smoking could conceivably be causative in either direction: perhaps persons with lung cancer were more inclined to smoke, so as to reduce pulmonary irritation caused by their cancers. Yet, Hill showed that most smokers began their habit in their youth, long before they developed lung cancer.

5. *Biological gradient*: This is the dose–response relationship – the more one smokes, the higher the rate of lung cancer. The presence of such a gradient allows one to identify a clear and often linear causative relationship. More complex nonlinear relationships can exist, however, such that again, this factor is not definitive, and its absence does not rule out causation.

6. *Plausibility*: It is helpful, writes Hill, if the causative inference is biologically plausible. This is a weak criterion, since "what is biologically plausible depends on the biological knowledge of the day" (Hill 1965, p. 298), which in turn often depends on the presence or absence of clinical/observational suggestions of topics for biological research. There is a vicious circle here: before Hill's work, since no one had raised seriously the association between cigarette smoking and lung cancer, biological researchers would not have been exposed to the idea that it should be studied. Thus, when Hill and his group identified the clinical association, they were faced with a biological abyss of nothingness – no biological research was available to explain their findings. Indeed, it took decades to come. Here is where Hill makes an important claim, which dates back to Hippocrates and which conflicts with many of the assumptions of biological researchers: clinical observation trumps biology, not vice versa. We should believe our clinical eyes, sharpened by the lenses of statistics and epidemiology; we should not reject what we see just because our biological theories do not yet explain it. Hill quotes the physician Arthur Conan's Doyle's wise medical advice, put in the mouth of Sherlock Holmes: "When you have eliminated the impossible, whatever remains, *however improbable*, must be the truth" (Hill 1965, p. 298).

7. *Coherence*: While one must be open to observations that await confirmation by biological research, we should also put our observations in the context of what is reasonably well proven biologically: "the cause-and-effect interpretation of our data should not seriously conflict with the generally known facts of the natural history and biology of the disease" (Hill 1965, p. 298). One would not want to invoke an extraterrestrial cause of medical disease, for instance. This is not altogether irrelevant: in recent years, a generally sane full professor of psychiatry at Harvard observed cases of persons with sexual trauma who attributed those events to alien abduction. After collecting a number of cases, the psychiatrist argued (in a nonscientifically peer-reviewed best-selling book) for a cause-and-effect relationship on standard scientific grounds (Mack 1995). Applying Hill's advice, there was an association: the effect size was there, it was consistent, apparently specific, obeyed temporality of cause and effect, and even appeared to have a dose-and-effect relationship (people who reported longer

periods of abduction experienced more posttraumatic-stress symptoms). But it was radically incoherent with the minimal facts of human biology.

Thus, coherence is not a minor matter, though it might seem somewhat trivial. If a proposed cause and effect relationship is illogical, it is a weak proposal; and many logical relationships are incoherent metaphysically.

8. *Experiment*: This is the whole of scientific causation outside of the world of human beings – that is, outside of clinical research. In basic research, with cells or animals or ions, one can conduct a true experiment. By holding all aspects of the environment stable except for one factor, one can definitively conclude that x causes y. With humans, this kind of environmental control is unethical and infeasible. In effect, RCTs are experiments with humans. They are how we can get at this aspect of causation, though again only with probability (albeit often quite high), not absolute certainty (unlike, perhaps, completely controlled animal experiments). Perhaps because he was speaking to epidemiologists rather than statisticians, Hill did not emphasize the role of RCTs as experiment in his address. Rather, he pointed out that sometimes we can make interventions that can help support causation: for instance, did the removal of an exposure prevent further cases of disease? This would support a causative relationship.

Perhaps Hill also downplayed the role of RCTs in experimentation because of his debate with Fisher. Fisher was saying that RCTs were a sine qua non of causation; Hill wanted to argue otherwise, partly because RCTs were unethical or infeasible for many important topics, such as cigarette smoking.

As a more general conceptual matter, I would tend to agree with Fisher, and I think we should be more definitive than Hill: I would not place experiment eighth on the list of causation; I would define it as meaning RCTs, *where feasible* (thus in agreement with Hill in regards to cigarette smoking), and I would place it first, because it gives us the strongest evidence (though, again, it is not definitive).

Recall that even here no criterion is essential. The absence of RCTs does not rule out causation, and its presence is not required to infer causation. Again, since this reflects human experimentation, questions of feasibility and ethics arise: No RCT ever demonstrated that cigarette smoking causes lung cancer, nor can or should it. We would have to randomize two large groups of people, probably with at least 5,000 in each arm, to smoke or not smoke for about 10–20 years, and then assess incurable lung cancer as the outcome. Enough said.

9. *Analogy*: This feature of causation deserves to be last since, like coherence, though it is relevant, it can be trivial. Hill notes that since rubella, for instance, is associated with pregnancy-related malformations, some other viruses can be expected to pose similar risks.

These are Hill's nine features of causation, given in the order of importance which he used. I would reorder them as noted in Table 14.1.

Often called the "Hill criteria," we should keep in mind that causation is not a matter of checklists and criteria; rather, it is a conceptual problem, as Hume demonstrated. And one needs to weight different features of the evidence, clinical and biological, in coming to conclusions regarding causation. Even with all this effort, as Hume pointed out long ago, causation is still usually a matter of a high level of probability, rather than absolute certainty (see next chapter).

Table 14.1 A. Bradford Hill's features of causation

1. Experiment (RCTs)

2. Strength of an association (effect size)

3. Consistency of an association (replication)

4. Specificity

5. Relationship in time (cause precedes effect)

6. Biological gradient (dose–response relationship)

7. Biological plausibility

8. Coherence of the evidence

9. Reasoning by analogy

RCTs = randomized clinical trials.
Adapted from Hill 1965.

Sir Richard Doll, Hill's younger associate, has suggested reducing this list to four key features, which, if met on a specific topic, should be definitive proof of causation:

> With the experience that we now have of thousands of epidemiological studies, we can conclude that large relative risks – on the order of >20:1 – with evidence of a dose-response relationship, that cannot be explained by methodological bias or reasonably be attributed to chance (with p-levels of $< 1 \times 10^{-6}$) are in themselves adequate proof of a causal relationship.
> (Doll 2002, p. 512)

Here are the four factors:

a)   a huge relative risk;
b)   a dose–response relationship;
c)   minimal bias; and
d)   tiny likelihood by chance (p < 0.00001).

Doll points out that the 1950 cigarette smoking data met these criteria; this is sobering, since a half century more had to pass before the force of this truth could overcome the power of the organized lies produced by the tobacco industry (proving the importance of the politics of research; see Chapter 17). It is also sobering, however, because Doll is arguing for agreement on a high threshold. Today, as he admits, most of our evidence falls far below this threshold – hence the need for attention to the other features identified by Hill. Thus, a small relative risk of cancer caused by estrogenic contraceptives can still be convincing when supplemented by animal studies demonstrating similar effects.

Biological Causation

We might contrast Hill's features of causation – which is the core of epidemiology and a conceptual linchpin for the evidence-based medicine (EBM) approach – with the traditional biological approach in medicine encapsulated in Koch's postulates for causation. In the beginning of the bacterial era, the nineteenth-century German physician Robert Koch argued that we could conclude that a bacterial agent caused a particular disease if the following postulates are met:

1. Whenever an agent was cultured, the disease was there.
2. Whenever the disease was not there, the agent could not be cultured.
3. When the agent was removed, the disease went away (Salsburg 2001a, p. 186).

As Salsburg points out, this definition of causation is similar to what the philosopher Bertrand Russell would later call "material implication" (see the next chapter). It can apply to some (though not all) infectious diseases in which the bacterial agent is *necessary and sufficient* to cause disease. Yet many causes are necessary but not sufficient; others are sufficient but not necessary. Some causes are neither necessary nor sufficient, but they are still causes. Cigarette smoking is in this last category: one can get lung cancer without smoking; one can smoke without getting lung cancer – but it is a cause. The biological definition of causation fails for most chronic medical illnesses that have more than one cause. This was the problem Hill was trying to solve.

Causation Is a Concept, Not a Number

Hill ended his discussion by reminding us that causation is not about chance and the use of statistics: it is a conceptual matter. Again, p-values and statistical significance are not relevant. This common misconception is such a major problem in medical statistics, in my view, that I wish to let Hill speak for himself on this matter, beckoning from 1965 to new generations of clinicians and researchers:

> "Between the two world wars there was a strong case for emphasizing to the clinician and other research workers the importance of not overlooking the play of chance upon their data. Perhaps too often generalities were based upon two men and a laboratory dog while the treatment of choice was deduced from a difference between two bedfuls of patients and might easily have not true meaning. It was therefore a useful corrective for statisticians to stress, and to teach the need for, tests of significance merely to serve as guides to caution before drawing a conclusion, before inflating the particular to the general.
>
> I wonder whether the pendulum has not swung too far – not only with the attentive pupils but even with the statisticians themselves. To decline to draw conclusions without standard errors can surely be just as silly? . . . [T]here are innumerable situations in which [tests of significance] are totally unnecessary – because the difference is grotesquely obvious, because it is negligible, or because, whether it be formally significant or not, it is too small to be of any practical importance. What is worse the glitter of the *t* table diverts attention from the inadequacies of the fare . . .
>
> Of course I exaggerate. Yet too often I suspect we waste a deal of time, we grasp the shadow and lose the substance, we weaken our capacity to interpret data and to take reasonable decisions whatever the value of P. And far too often we deduce "no difference" from "no significant difference." Like fire, the χ^2 test is an excellent servant and a bad master."
>
> (Hill 1965, pp. 299–300)

Practical Causation

A final point is in order, one on which Hill ends his address: Causation is not a theoretical matter for medicine; it is a practical one. The reason I infer, or do not infer, causation is because I will, or will not, give drug X to patient Y. The threshold for inferring causation may differ depending on the practical matter at hand. If I am thinking of giving a drug with major toxicities, I will want many, if not most, of Hill's features to be met. If I am the Surgeon General and I am thinking of restricting the civil rights of citizens to smoke in restaurants, I will want many, if not most, of Hill's features to be met. However, if I am a researcher inferring causation on a matter of little practical importance (e.g., that sunlight exposure decreases latency to REM sleep), a lower threshold for acceptance of causation will not harm anyone. The truth will remain the truth wherever we put our thresholds for causation, but we should not immobilize ourselves when important practical questions need to be answered (Bayesian statistics provides a way to manage this problem; see Chapter 13). We still need to decide, one way or the other, and *not* deciding, as the philosopher William James reminded us so well, is one way of deciding (the easy, passive way) (James 1956 [1897]). Recall that statistics is not meant to keep us from inferring causation, or doing something, because we are not absolutely, or near absolutely, certain. Statistics is merely a way, as La Place put it, of quantifying, rather than ignoring, error. How much error we are willing to accept depends on the circumstances. Here is Hill:

> [O]n relatively slight evidence we might decide to restrict the use of a drug for early-morning sickness in pregnant women. If we are wrong in deducing causation from association no great harm will be done. The good lady and the pharmaceutical industry will doubtless survive . . . All scientific work is incomplete – whether it be observational or experimental. All scientific work is liable to be upset or modified by advancing knowledge. That does not confer upon us a freedom to ignore the knowledge we already have, or to postpone the action that it appears to demand at a given time.
>
> Who knows, asked Robert Browning, but the world may end tonight? True, but on available evidence most of us make ready to commute on the 8.30 next day.
>
> (Hill 1965, p. 300)

Replication and the Wish to Believe

To this point, readers will be aware that if statistics are well understood, both conceptually and historically, no single report can be seen as definitive. Replication is a key feature for attributing causation to any medical claim. If nothing else, the cigarette smoking and lung cancer controversy between Fisher and Hill should have taught us this fact. History is poorly studied, however, and statistics are little understood conceptually.

As a result, it seems to be the case that first impressions, from initial studies or early reports, have staying power in the consciousness of clinicians.

This phenomenon has begun to be documented empirically. In one analysis (Ioannidis 2005), researchers examined 49 highly cited original clinical research studies, most of which claimed benefit with a treatment. Later studies contradicted the initial findings in 16%, or found a smaller effect size of benefit in another 16%; 44% were replicated; and 24% were never re-examined. Initial reports were more likely to be later contradicted if they were nonrandomized (5/6, 83%, of nonrandomized studies were contradicted versus only 9/39, 23%, of RCTs), or if they were randomized but small in sample size.

If we apply Hill's feature of replication, more than half of highly cited clinical research studies fail the test. This would be enough to give us pause if it were not the case that it seems that clinicians and researchers appear to more readily accept positive than negative replication. Clinical opinions persist, even after they have been studied and refuted (Tatsioni, Bonitsis, and Ioannidis 2007). Tatsioni and colleagues examined the view that vitamin

E supplementation has cardiovascular benefits, a perspective fostered by reports from large epidemiological studies in 1993. Other nonrandomized studies also found benefit, as did one RCT in 2002. But the largest and best-designed study found no benefit in 2000, and a meta-analysis of all these studies in 2004 also found no benefit, instead finding increased risk of death at high vitamin E doses. The authors analyzed studies published in the year 1997, so that they were written before most of the RCTs, compared to later articles in 2005 after the publication of clear contradiction of the initial hypothesis of benefit. Although articles written in 1997 were much less unfavorable (2%) to vitamin E than articles written in 2005 (34%), the authors noted that 50% of articles in 2005 continued to favorably cite the earlier literature, by then disproven. They found similar patterns with initial studies of benefit, later disproven, with beta-carotene for cancer and estrogen for dementia.

The researchers noted that specialty, more so than generalist, journals tended to continue to publish favorable articles about the disproven treatments. They also observed that

> In the evaluation of counterarguments, we encountered almost any source of bias, genuine diversity, and biological reasoning invoked to defend the original observations . . . consistent with a belief that is defended at all cost. The defense of the observations was persistent, despite the availability of very strong contradicting randomized evidence on the same topic. Thus, one wonders whether any contradicted associations may ever be entirely abandoned . . . For most associations and questions of medical interest, either no randomized data exist, or the randomized evidence is minimal and of poor quality.
>
> (Tatsioni, Bonitsis, and Ioannidis 2007, p. 2525)

Though perhaps disappointed, a half century after their debates, I do not think Hill and Fisher would be surprised.

Chapter 15

A Philosophy of Statistics

Truth is corrected error.

(Charles Sanders Peirce) (Peirce 1958b)

Statistics, as a discipline, does not exist in a vacuum. It is a reflection of our views on science, and thus how it is understood and how it is used depends on what we mean by "science." Most statistics texts do not discuss these matters or, if they do, they are perfunctory. But it is important for all involved (statisticians and clinicians) to appreciate their assumptions, and to have some rationale for them.

Cultural Positivism

Most doctors and clinicians have an unconscious philosophy of science, imbibed from the larger culture: positivism. Positivism is the view that science is the accumulation of facts. Fact upon fact produces scientific laws. Holding sway through much of the nineteenth and twentieth centuries, the positivistic view of science has seeped into our bones. Beginning in the late nineteenth century, and more definitely after the 1960s, philosophers of science have shown that "facts" do not exist as independent entities; they are tied to theories and hypotheses. Facts cannot be separated from theories; science involves deduction, not just induction.

The nineteenth-century American philosopher Charles Sanders Peirce, who was a practicing physicist, knew what was involved in the actual practice of science: The scientist has a hypothesis, a theory; this theory might have been based on previous studies, or it might simply be imagined wholecloth (Peirce called this "abduction"); the scientist then tries to verify or refute his theory by facts (either passively, through observation, or actively, through experiment). In this way, no facts are observed without a preceding hypothesis. So facts are "theory-laden"; between fact and theory no sharp line can be drawn (Jaspers 1997 [1959]).

Verify or Refute?

This hypothesis–fact relationship leaves us with a dilemma: in testing our hypotheses, which is more important: verification or refutation? The positivistic view was biased in favor of confirming theories: fact was placed upon fact to verify theories (another name for this view of science is "verificationism"). In the mid-twentieth century, Karl Popper rejected positivism by privileging refutation over confirmation: a single negative result was definitive – it refuted an hypothesis – while any positive result was always provisional – it never definitively proves a hypothesis, because it can always be refuted by a negative result. Let us examine Popper's views, and how they apply to different approaches to statistics, more closely.

Karl Popper's Philosophy of Science

I think it would be fair to argue that in today's world of science and medical research, the assumed philosophy of science (sometimes explicit) is that of the philosopher Karl Popper (Popper 1959). Popper sought to provide a deductive definition of science to replace the more traditional inductive definition. In the older view, science seemed to involve the accumulation of facts; the more facts, the more science. The problem with this inductive view can be traced back to David Hume, who showed that this approach could never, with complete certainty, prove anything (see the previous chapter). Popper sought complete certainty for science, and he thought he had it with Einstein's discoveries. Einstein was able to make certain predictions based on his theories; if those predictions were wrong, then his theory was wrong. Only one mistake was required to disprove his entire theory. Popper argued that science could best be understood as an activity whose theories could be definitively disproven, but never definitively proven. The best scientific theories, then, would be those which would make falsifiable propositions and, if not falsified, then those theories might be true. Popper specified Freud and Marx for blame for having claimed to provide scientific theories when in fact their ideas were in no way falsifiable. This approach has become quite popular among modern scientists. It has the disadvantage, however, of taking one part of science. Freud and Marx are, in some sense, easy targets; Darwin's theory could just as well be rejected for being unfalsifiable. Ultimately, Popper did not solve the Humean riddle, for Popper's view tells us not which theories are true, but which ones are not.

The Limits of Refutation

We might summarize that contemporary views of science (heavily influenced by Popper) are focused on hypothesis testing by refutation. We see this philosophy reflected in statistics, especially in the whole concept of the importance of the p-value and the idea of trying to refute the null hypothesis (see Chapter 7).

My own view is that this refutationism is as wrong as the old verificationism, because no single refutation is definitive. One can have positive results after negative results; what, then, to make of the original negative results? In statistics, this overemphasis on refutation leads to overuse of p-values, while appropriate appreciation of positive results would lead us to a different kind of statistics (descriptive effect size oriented methods; see Chapter 9).

Charles Peirce's Philosophy of Science

This leads to an inductive philosophy of science, like that of Charles Peirce (Peirce 1958a), but not exactly in the traditional sense. Peirce accepted induction as the method of science, acknowledged that it led to increasing probabilities of truth, and argued that these probabilities reached the limits of certainty so closely that it was mathematically meaningless to deny certainty to them at a certain point of accumulated evidence. Peirce also added that this accumulation of near-certain inductive knowledge was a process that spanned generations of scientists and that the community of scientists which added to this fund of knowledge would eventually reach consensus on what was likely to be true based on those data.

Causation Again

We can now return to that key philosophical aspect of statistics: the problem of causation. In the previous chapter, I reviewed the basic idea of the eighteenth-century philosopher David Hume, arguing that inductive inference did not lead to absolute certainty of causation. The philosopher Bertrand Russell tried to provide another way of looking at the question with his notion of "material implication." Russell argued that if A causes B, we are saying that A "materially implies" B. In other words, there is something in A that is also entailed in B (Salsburg 2001a). He distinguished this material implication from the symbolic nature of other logical relationships (such as conjunction – the "and" relationship – or disjunction – the "or" relationship). When we say "if A, then B," the "if, then" relationship is not purely symbolic, but has some material basis. This was Russell's view; it does not solve the problem of causation, but it suggests a way of thinking about causation that entails that the idea is not a matter of purely symbolic logic, but perhaps an empirical matter.

A final way of thinking about causation – besides Hume's description of induction, and Russell's logical concept of material implication – is a scientific perspective that can be traced to one of the French founders of nineteenth-century experimental medicine, Claude Bernard (Olmsted 1952). Bernard held that we could conclude that A causes B by conducting an experiment in which all conditions are held constant except A, and showing that B follows. Such proof of causation is based on being able to control all factors except one, the experimental factor. This is, in practice, difficult to do in biology and medicine, and much more feasible in inorganic sciences such as physics and chemistry. But it can be done. For instance, we have the technology today to conduct animal studies in which the entire animal genome is fixed beforehand; animals can be genetically bred to produce a certain genetic state and they can all be identical in that genetic state; we can then control the animals' environment from birth until death. In that kind of controlled setting, where all genetic and environmental factors are controlled, Bernard's definition of experimental causation may hold.

Such causation is unethical and infeasible with human beings. The closest we get to it is with randomization. As discussed throughout this book, randomization with human beings, though reducing much uncertainty, never reduces all uncertainty, and thus we cannot achieve absolute causation. The importance of RCTs in getting us very much closer to causation might be highlighted by realizing that they are the closest human approximation to Bernard's *experimental causation*. Fisher was right in emphasizing the need for RCTs in asserting causation, and Hill was right in recognizing the benefits of other features of research, in addition to experimentation with RCTs, so as to reduce uncertainty even further.

The General Versus the Individual

Another philosophical aspect of statistics is how it reflects the general as opposed to the individual. The Belgian thinker Quetelet recognized the issue in the 1840s; he "knew that individuals' characteristics could not be represented by a deterministic law, but he believed that averages over groups could be so represented" (Stigler 1986, p. 172). About half a century later, two German philosophers, Wilhelm Windelband and Heinrich Rickert, made this general distinction the basis for their understanding of the nature and limits of science: Science consists of general laws; it stops short of the unique and the individual. They said there were two kinds of knowledge: nosographic (general, statistical, group-based) and idiographic (individual and unique for each particular case). Science "explained" (*Erklaren*) general laws; philosophy and the humanities "understood" (*Verstehen*) the unique characteristics of individuals (Makkreel 1992).

This criticism of statistics, so often used by modern critics of evidence-based medicine (EBM), was present from the very beginning of the effort (in the mid-nineteenth century) to apply statistics to human beings (as in experimental psychology), as opposed to limiting it to mathematics, astronomy, and physics (as had previously been the case). Here is an example from Auguste Comte, attacking the statistician Poisson, who in 1835 had suggested there might be legal uses for statistics: "The application of this calculus to matters of morality is repugnant to the soul. It amounts, for example, to representing the truth of a verdict by a number, to thus treat men as if they were dice, each with many faces, some for error, some for truth" (Stigler 1986, p. 194).

This history reminds me of an exchange I recently had, one that became somewhat heated, during a symposium at the annual convention of the American Psychiatric Association. I and others had reviewed RCTs showing that antidepressants were hardly effective in bipolar depression; one of the discussants, who had previously supported their use, had to bow to the data, but he ended his presentation by declaring forcefully: "Antidepressants may not be as great as we had hoped, but, in the end, your individual experience as a practitioner and that of the patient trumps everything!" Raucous applause followed from the packed audience of clinicians. Fearing that three hours of painstaking exposition of RCT data had just been flushed down a toilet, and perhaps angry about such dismissal of years of daily effort by researchers like me, I wanted to retort: "Only if you don't care about science." But a debate about philosophy of science could not occur then and there.

This is the problem: Yes, statistics do not tell you what to do with the individual case, but this does not mean that a clinician should decide what to do out of thin air. The clinician's decisions about the individual case need to be *informed*, not *dictated*, by scientific knowledge as established in a general way through statistics.

This insight is present in the great neo-Hippocratic thinkers of modern medicine. Perhaps the best example is William Osler, who always emphasized that medicine was not just a science but also an art, and that "the art of medicine is the art of balancing probabilities" (Osler 1948). If we use the reality of art to negate the necessity of science, we might as well start Galenic bleeding all over again. The art of medicine is, in fact, as Osler suggests, the proper appreciation of the science via a knowledge of statistics: *the art of balancing probabilities*.

The problem with that leader's comment was that he was *negating* the general knowledge of statistics by prioritizing the individual experience of clinicians. The history of medicine, and a rational approach to the philosophy of science, indicates that the prioritization should be the other way around (which is the basic perspective of EBM).

The Illogic of Hypothesis-Testing Statistics

The key philosophical problem of statistics is perhaps the problem of induction, as described earlier. At a practical level, hypothesis-testing statistics, as we currently use them, suffer from faulty probability logic, as I described in Chapter 7. It is worth explaining the importance of this invalid logic in more detail.

Logic, as a branch of philosophy, examines whether one's conclusions flow from one's premises. In philosophy, logic is seen as an important method because, no matter what the content of one's views, if the logical structure of an argument is invalid, then the whole argument is faulty. We may or may not agree with the content of any statement (the world is round; the world is flat), but we should all be able to agree on the logic of any claim that if x is true, then y must be true. If an argument is illogical, then it can simply be dismissed.

This is the basic perspective of most contemporary philosophy. Usually logic refers to "predicate" logic, meaning discussions of statements about present facts: things that are. However, what may be true in *predicate* logic – things that *are* – is not always true for other kinds of logic, such as *modal* logic – things that *necessarily* are – and *probability* logic – things that *probably* are. Cohen had the intuition that the key problem of hypothesis-testing statistics is that it is based on a structure that *works in predicate logic, but fails in probability logic.*

Predicate logic applied to hypothesis testing statistics would be as follows:

"If the null hypothesis [NH] is correct, then these data *cannot occur.*
These data have occurred.
Therefore, the null hypothesis *is false.*"

This argument is logically valid, but it becomes invalid once it is turned into a statement of probability:

"If the null hypothesis [NH] is correct, then these data *are highly unlikely.*
These data have occurred.
Therefore, the null hypothesis *is highly unlikely.*"

I have italicized the differences where we have moved from statements of fact to statements of probability. The falsity of this transition becomes clear once we use examples. Using predicate logic:

"If a person is a Martian, then he is not a member of Congress.
This person is a member of Congress.
Therefore, he is not a Martian."
This logic of facts is valid; but the logic of probability is invalid:
"If a person is an American then he is probably not a member of Congress.
This person is a member of Congress.

Therefore, he is probably not American." (Pollard and Richardson 1987)

Cohen calls this logical fallacy "the illusion of attaining improbability," and if true, which appears to be the case, it undercuts the very basis of hypothesis-testing statistics and, thereby, the vast majority of medical research. The whole industry of p-values comes tumbling down.

Inductive Logic

Medical statistics are based on observation, and thus they are a species of induction. Induction, in turn, is philosophically complex. It turns out that one cannot easily infer causation from observation, and that the logic of our hypothesis-testing methods is faulty. What are we to do?

Once again, the answer seems to be to give up our theories and return more closely to our observation. The more we engage in descriptive statistics, the farther away we get from hypothesis-mongering, the closer we are to a conceptually sound use of statistics. We can quantitate without minimal speculating.

I hope some day to be able to publish research studies on small sample sizes where the results can be accepted as they are, with the main limitation of imprecision, but without the irrelevant claim that they can only be "hypothesis-generating" as opposed to "hypothesis-testing." Science is not about hypothesis-testing or hypothesis-generating; it is about the complex interrelation between theory and fact, and the gradual accumulation of evidence for or against any scientific hypothesis. Perhaps we can then get beyond the logical fallacies so rampant in statistical debates, so closely related to the lament of a philosopher: "All logic texts are divided into two parts. In the first part, on deductive logic, the fallacies are explained; in the second part, on inductive logic, they are committed" (Cohen 1994).

Evidence-Based Medicine: Defense and Criticism

There is a case to be made for evidence-based medicine (EBM), and there is a case to be made against it. Many of the critiques of EBM are, I believe, ill-founded, but there are some important criticisms that need attention. Recently, for example, prominent biologically oriented senior figures in psychiatry have published provocative papers in critique of EBM as applied to psychiatry (Levine and Fink 2006). They argue that EBM can only be applied to psychiatry if three assumptions hold: "Is the diagnostic system valid? Are the data from clinical trials assessing efficacy and safety valid? Are they in a form that can be applied to clinical practice?" (Levine and Fink 2006, p. 402). The authors then negatively on all three fronts, highlighting the limitations of the DSM-IV psychiatric nosology, referring to misconduct in the practice of clinical trials (e.g., inclusion of borderline qualifying patients), and emphasizing how the pharmaceutical industry misuses clinical trials for its own economic purposes. Others have appropriately emphasized the importance of the humanities, as opposed to just EBM, in psychiatry (Bolwig 2006). And still others note the persistence of authority ("eminence-based medicine") as a key aspect of psychiatric practice, suggesting that EBM cannot replace it (Stahl 2002). Despite some attempts in the psychiatric literature (Soldani, Ghaemi, and Baldessarini 2005) to clarify the uses of EBM, as well as its limits, there still seems to be mistrust about the EBM approach among many psychiatrists.

Here, I will make the case for EBM, and then we can see its limitations. The context I will use relates to psychiatry, but most of the same issues apply to all of medicine.

The History of Non-EBM

Both in name and as a movement, EBM is only a few decades old; but as a concept it is ancient, and thus to appreciate it one must begin long ago.

In the fifth century AD, a brilliant physician had a powerful idea: the four humors, in varied combinations, produced all illness. From that date until a century ago, Galen's theory ruled medicine. Its corollary was that the treatment of disease involved getting the humors back in order; releasing them through bloodletting was the most common procedure, often augmented by other means of freeing bodily fluids (e.g., purgatives and laxatives). For 14 centuries, physicians subscribed to this wondrous biological theory of disease: we bled our patients until they lost their entire blood supply; we forced them to puke and defecate and urinate; we alternated extremely hot showers with extremely frigid ones – all in the name of normalizing those humors (Porter 1997). It all proved to be wrong.

This is not a "Whiggish" (or progressive) interpretation of history; it is not simply a matter of "they were wrong and we are right." Galen, Avicenna, Benjamin Rush – these were far more intelligent and creative men than we are. Not only am I not Whiggish,

I believe we are repeating these past errors: 14 centuries of ignorance have sunk deep marks into the flesh of the medical profession. As Sir George Pickering, Regius Professor of Medicine at Oxford, said in 1949:

> Modern medicine still preserves much of the attitude of mind of the school men of the Middle Ages. It tends to be omniscient rather than admit ignorance, to encourage speculation not solidly backed by evidence, and to be indifferent to the proof or disproof of hypothesis. It is to this legacy of the Middle Ages that may be attributed the phenomenon . . . (of) "the mysterious viability of the false."
>
> (Pickering 1949, p. 230–1)

We see this influence even today in such articles as the aforementioned critique of EBM as applied to psychiatry. I will be repeating some notions described in other chapters, but this repetition is meant to solidify in the reader's mind the importance of such concepts. Let us review the scientific and conceptual rationale for statistics in general, and for EBM in particular.

Galen Versus Hippocrates

There are, and always have been, two basic philosophies of medicine. One is *Galenic*: There is a theory, and it is right. For our purposes, the content of such theories do not matter (they can be about humors, serotonin and dopamine neurotransmitters [Stahl 2005], ECT [Fink and Taylor 2007], or even psychoanalysis): what matters is that hardly any scientific theory (especially in medicine) is absolutely right (Ghaemi 2003). The error is not so much in the content, but in the method of this way of thinking: the focus is on theory, not reality; on beliefs, not facts; on concepts, not clinical observations. If the facts do not agree with the theory, so much the worse for the facts. This perspective led Galen to think that if patients did not respond to his treatments, they were ipso facto incurable (shades of notions such as "treatment-resistant depression"):

> All who drink of this treatment recover in a short time,
> Except those whom it does not help, who all die.
> It is obvious, therefore, that it fails only in incurable cases.
>
> (Galen, quoted in Silverman 1998, p. 3)

There is, and has always been, a second approach, much more humble and simple – the idea that clinical observation, first and foremost, should precede any theory; that theories should be sacrificed to observations, and not vice versa; that clinical realities are more basic than any other theory; and that treatments should also be based on observational bases, not ideas. This second approach was first promulgated clearly by *Hippocrates* and his school in the fifth century BC, but Galen demolished Hippocratic medicine (while claiming its mantle) and it lay dormant until revived 1,000 years later in the Renaissance (McHugh 1996; Ghaemi 2008).

Hippocratic Humility

Why all this historical background in a discussion of EBM? Because it is important to know what the options are, and what the stakes. Either we are Hippocratic or we are Galenic; either we value clinical observation or we value theories. The debate comes down to this.

If readers, including EBM critics, claim that they value clinical observation, then the question is: How can we validate clinical observation? How do we know when our observations are correct and when they are false?

Readers of this book will recognize that the core problem is *confounding bias* (Miettinen and Cook 1981), a deep and very basic clinical problem: *we, clinicians, cannot believe our eyes*. It can appear that something is the case when it is not; that some treatment is improving matters when it is not. These confounding factors are present not just some of the time, but *most* of the time.

Perhaps most clinicians would admit this basic fact, but it is important to draw both the *clinical* and *scientific* implications.

Clinically, the reality of confounding bias teaches us the deep need for a Hippocratic humility, as opposed to a Galenic arrogance (Galen once said: "My treatment only fails in incurable cases") – a recognition that we might be wrong, indeed we often are, even in our most definitive clinical experiences (Ghaemi 2008). Everybody thought Galen was right for 14 centuries; the end of Galenic treatments came about in the nineteenth century *because of* EBM – "the numerical method" of Pierre Louis (Porter 1997). *Counting patients*, the numerical method, EBM – that has been the source of the greatest medical advances, not the exquisite case study, nor the brilliance of any one person (be he Freud or Kraepelin or even our most prominent professors today), nor decades of clinical experience. Hill noted that the common distinction between clinical experience and clinical research is a false one (Hill 1962a): after all, clinical experience is based on the recollection of cases, usually a few cases; clinical research is simply the claim that such recollection is biased, and that the remedy is to collect more than just a few cases, *and* to compare them in ways that reduce bias. The latter point entails EBM.

Truths of theory are transient. Not only is Galen out of date, but so is the much vaunted catecholamine theory of depression; today's most sophisticated neurobiology will be passé by the end of the decade. Clinical observation and research, in contrast, is more steady: That same melancholia that Hippocrates described can be discerned in today's major depression; that same mania that Arateus of Cappadocia explained in the second century AD is visible in current mania. (Obviously, social and cultural factors come into play, and such presentations vary somewhat in different epochs, as social constructionists will point out; Foucault 1994.) Clinical research is the solid ground of medicine; biological theory is a necessary but changing superstructure. If these relations are reversed, then mere speculation takes over and the more solid ground of science is lost.

Scientifically, confounding bias leads to the conclusion that *any* observation, even the most repeated and detailed, can be – indeed, often is – wrong; thus, valid clinical judgments can only be made after removing confounding factors (Miettinen and Cook 1981; Rothman and Greenland 1998).

Randomization, as discussed throughout this book, is the most effective way to remove confounding bias, and it has disproven many widely accepted treatments that proved to be ineffective, harmful, or both.

If we accept, then, that clinical observation is the core of medicine (rather than theory), and that confounding bias afflicts it, and that randomization is the best solution, then we have accepted EBM. That is the core of EBM, and the rationale for the levels of evidence where randomized data are more valid than observational data (Soldani, Ghaemi, and Baldessarini 2005). These are new methods, and the major advances in medical treatment of the past 50 years are unimaginable without RCTs specifically, and EBM more generally.

Indeed, perhaps the greatest public health advance of our era – the linking of cigarette smoking and cancer (led by Hill) – was both source and consequence of EBM methods. As to the relevance of EBM to psychiatry, after the streptomycin RCT, among the first RCTs to happen were in psychiatry, with chlorpromazine and lithium in the early 1950s (Healy 2001).

Psychiatric Nosology

Critics of EBM often make much of the limitations of psychiatric nosology (Levine and Fink 2006). Yet EBM has little to do with diagnosis. EBM, as formally advanced in recent years (Sackett et al. 2000), has mainly had to do with treatment, not diagnosis; it focuses on treatment studies, on randomization (which is only relevant to treatment, not diagnosis), and on such statistical techniques that relate to treatment (like meta-analysis, number needed to treat, etc.) (Sackett et al. 2000). Validating diagnoses is a matter for another field (clinical epidemiology) (Robins and Guze 1970; Ghaemi 2003). (To the extent that diagnosis is addressed at all in most of the EBM literature, it has to do with subjects like the sensitivity and specificity of diagnostic tests, the classic example being V/Q scans for deep venous thrombosis [Jaeschke, Guyatt, and Sackett 1994], not theoretical questions about etiology of illnesses or diagnostic criteria.) One could define schizophrenia in a completely opposite manner, as DSM-5 does; assessments of treatment would still need to account for confounding bias, and the consequent validity of RCTs would still hold.

One can be, not unjustifiably, fed up with DSM-5 and its impact on contemporary psychiatry, but there is no rationale in blaming EBM for it. We are dealing with the true (DSM-5 is mostly false), true (EBM has limitations), and unrelated (they have nothing to do with each other).

The Pharmaceutical Industry

The same perspective holds for critiques of how RCTs are designed and conducted, and how they are influenced by the pharmaceutical industry. None of this gets at the core rationale for EBM. Indeed, for-profit research groups can conduct clinical research invalidly and unethically, as can pharmaceutical companies; but the same could be said about the private practice of medicine, which can be conducted unethically and yet does not invalidate clinical medicine as such. Evidence-based medicine is not invalidated based on details about how clinical trials are run; randomized trials can still be faulty for many reasons (dropouts can be high, inclusion and exclusion criteria can be wrong, and so on) (Friedman, Furberg, and DeMets 1998a). But, again, this only means that those studies need to be conducted correctly, not incorrectly. The core rationale for randomized clinical trials (to remove confounding bias) remains unaffected.

Anti-Statistics Bias

There is, I believe, a general anti-statistics bias among many critics of EBM, and this bias has existed since the 1800s, from the first attempts of Pierre Louis or Quetelet to apply statistics to any human activity. Some critics seem to have an unconscious libertarian streak, as if statistics removes the soul from humanity and deprives individuals of free will. Others come at the issue from a Galenic view of medicine, as if biological theories should trump clinical observations, or, alternatively, clinical observations alone – a statistical accumulation of numbers – are meaningless if not biologically explained. (These critics call this the "medical," as opposed to the statistical, approach to EBM; Fink and Taylor 2008.)

These critics would do well to re-examine that primal medical controversy: cigarette smoking and lung cancer. As discussed previously, the importance of medical statistics grew out of, and was proven by, this controversy. This is a matter that has been well documented historically (Parascandola 2004). Medicine, like politics, involves a great deal of moral responsibility because human lives are in play. How many lives were lost over half a century of indecision, partly due to an ill-informed attack on statistics by biologically oriented physicians? Critics of EBM need to keep this history in mind.

The Cult of the Swan-Ganz Catheter

Nor need one go back far in history. We have good examples today of the hazards of this apparently hard-nosed "biological" approach to medicine, disparaging clinical research and statistical methods. A great example is the Swan-Ganz catheter, a staple of coronary intensive care units throughout the 1980s and 1990s. I recall, as a medical intern in 1990, how much ritual was involved with the use of the Swan: dialing some of the treatments up, others down, getting moment-by-moment blood pressure readings. It all seemed as scientific as could possibly be. But it was all untested by clinical research methods, and, now disproven by RCTs, it has proven to be a farce, and a deadly one, since the placement of the catheter in the neck was a complicated and dangerous procedure. Despite a warning article in 1985 by a medical leader, "The cult of the Swan-Ganz catheter" (Robin 1985), clinicians went along with aggressively using it. As one physician describes now, looking back:

> Those of us in the cult of the Swan-Ganz catheter had many motivations to join: true belief based on experience or (less likely) research studies, economic interest, a desire to give our patients what is now called "standard of care," frustration at our lack of effective treatments, the need to feel that we were helping, the need to impress our attendings, or laziness.
>
> (Blank 2006, p. 1041)

Without EBM, all of medicine approximates a cult, with charismatic leaders and passionate followers. The dangers of a cult of medicine, however, are that not only are minds at risk, but so are bodies.

Ivory-Tower EBM

This is my defense of EBM, but I believe it deserves criticism as well, just different critiques than those already raised.

I think the most important but underappreciated misuse is what might be called *ivory-tower EBM* – the idea that unless there are double-blind randomized placebo-controlled data, then there *is* no "evidence" (Soldani, Ghaemi, and Baldessarini 2005). But there is always evidence: that is the whole point of EBM – to give us a method whereby we can weight that evidence. Even nonrandomized evidence may be correct and useful (in the absence of randomized data or given certain constraints; for instance, the link between cigarettes and smoking is completely based on nonrandomized evidence, but with a great deal of careful statistical analysis to assess confounding factors). This view reflects a rarefied positivism that reflects a lack of understanding of the nature of evidence (and science) (Soldani, Ghaemi, and Baldessarini 2005). In my experience as a researcher and author, it is not uncommon to hear academic leaders (and journal peer reviewers) disparage important observational data as mere "chart reviews," as if they are thereby useless. This is the dogma of the cost-cutters, be they insurance companies or even national governments. This kind of fetishization of RCTs reflects a misunderstanding of science. We need informed critiques of EBM – because it can be misunderstood, and even abused – not to destroy but, rather, to improve it.

Back to Galen

It is an irony of history, but the whole development of medical statistics can be seen as an attempt to end the Galenic tyranny of theory, an effort to end medical dogmatism, a wish to exalt the simple virtues of Hippocratic observation. Ivory-tower EBM brings us back to Galen, the purveyor of medical dogmatism, the ogre which Louis and Fisher and Hill had tried to slay through the development of medical statistics. Now, ironically, the peak of statistical activism, EBM run amuck, threatens to bring back the sacrifice of observations to theory.

Among the limitations of EBM, the medical epidemiologist Alvan Feinstein (Feinstein 1977) emphasizes the problem of the "average patient": the fact that RCTs produce average results for a homogeneous sample, rather than showing effects in clinically relevant sub-types. The clinician treats an old man, or a young girl, but the average of those two persons is a middle-aged hermaphrodite. The clinical trial, even if valid internally, just does not directly generalize to the individual patient seen by a clinician. This problem goes beyond generalizability and brings us back to the conceptual problem of the individual versus the general, as discussed in the previous chapter. The fetishization of RCTs reaches its climax, he argued (Feinstein and Horwitz 1997), in the Cochrane Collaboration, the "industrial scale" application of meta-analysis to determine the "best" available evidence (see Chapter 12). The Cochrane database completely ignores all observational studies, and thus it would not include any "evidence" that penicillin is effective. Hence, any attempt to claim "authoritative evidence," especially a methodology that would ignore penicillin, should raise our suspicion, Feinstein concludes. Such authoritarian claims, especially when manipulated in meta-analysis, can easily be abused, and then "a new form of dogmatic authoritarianism may then be revived in modern medicine, but the pronouncements will come from Cochranian Oxford rather than Galenic Rome" (Feinstein and Horwitz 1997, p. 535).

Parachutes for Gravitational Challenge

Bradford Hill noted that RCTs were unnecessary in certain cases; sometimes the effect of a treatment is so massive that its benefits are obvious: an example is penicillin. Sometimes, the disease is invariably fatal, so any benefit seen can be taken as real; Hill used the example of miliary or meningeal tuberculosis, invariably fatal conditions in contrast to pulmonary tuberculosis, which has a variable course. It is precisely in such variable conditions, Hill argued, that RCTs are needed. He was able to convince British authorities to allow the 1948 RCT of streptomycin for pulmonary, but not miliary or meningeal, tuberculosis on this rationale (Silverman 1998).

Many proponents of ivory-tower EBM do not appreciate Hill's insight: RCTs are not needed when outcomes are invariable.

This reality, so obvious to common sense but opaque to those who have become EBM true believers, was acknowledged by the *British Journal of Medicine*, which published a tongue-in-cheek article (written by obstetricians at Cambridge University in the United Kingdom) entitled "Parachute use to prevent death and major trauma related to gravitational challenge: Systematic review of randomized, controlled trials." The authors reported, after searching Medline, Web of Science, Embase, and the Cochrane library databases: "We were unable to identify any randomized controlled trials of parachute intervention" (Smith and Pell 2003, p. 1459). They noted that "the basis for parachute use is purely observational," and that the role of bias could not be discounted because "individuals jumping from aircraft without the help of a parachute are likely to have a high prevalence of pre-existing psychiatric morbidity and may also differ in key demographic factors, such as income and cigarette use. It follows, therefore, that the apparent protective effect of parachutes may be merely an example of the 'healthy cohort' effect" (Smith and Pell 2003, p. 1459). They noted that no "multivariate analytical approaches" had tried to correct for these biases. They also decried the use of parachutes as just another example of disease-mongering (see Chapter 17), "the medicalisation of free fall": "It might be argued that the pressure exerted on individuals to use parachutes is yet another example of a natural, life enhancing experience being turned into a situation of fear and dependency" (Smith and Pell 2003, p. 1459). Economic factors could not be ignored (see Chapter 17): "The parachute industry has earned billions of dollars for vast multinational corporations whose profits depend on belief in the efficacy of their product. One would hardly expect these vast commercial concerns to have the bravery to test their product in the setting of a randomized controlled trial." They conclude: "Individuals who insist that all interventions need to be validated by a randomized controlled trial need to come down to earth with a bump" (Smith and Pell 2003, p. 1460).

The Earth is Round (p < 0.05)

Another way of looking at the limitations of EBM is to realize that EBM is less applicable where quantitative methods are irrelevant or inapplicable. The statistician Jacob Cohen emphasized the limitations of medical statistics, the basis for EBM, with the above title to one of his papers (Cohen 1994).

As described in Chapter 11, the work of science is not about definitively proving or disproving any theory with any single study. "Facts" do not exist separate from theories, and thus scientific hypotheses are always only partially proven or disproven by specific studies. The convergence of replicated research, gradually approximating the truth (as Peirce described), is how science works. No p-value, and no RCT (and no meta-analysis), captures that convergence. For a long time, the world's consensus was that the world was flat. Over time, the consensus changed to the world being round. There are good grounds for this change, but they have nothing to do with p-values.

Appreciating, Not Abusing, EBM

Those who think EBM cannot be applied to psychiatry or medicine should think about the implications given the history of medicine. Without the application of scientific principles to clinical research, we will have nothing but opinion – a postmodern relativist world where all is ideology. Without scientific, evidence-based clinical research, in the Hippocratic tradition of careful attention to clinical observation – and its statistical correlates in the need for combating confounding bias – psychiatry, and all of medicine, would be but a mere shadow of what it is, and a pale reflection of what it can be. Not only should EBM be applied to psychiatry, but, if it is not, we will just go back to the brackish dogmatisms of the past, a return to the non-Hippocratic approach to medicine which failed humanity for so long. Two millennia are long enough to test a theory.

On the other hand, let us not make a fetish out of RCTs. Recall cigarettes once more: many important features of human disease cannot be settled by RCTs. EBM means *levels* of evidence, and a recognition of the *limits* of statistics (as well as their uses); not an ivory-tower positivism, an idealization of all-powerful placebo-based data, standing as absolute Truth; not a tool to be used for political or economic purposes – a fetish of governments, a profit-making plan for insurance companies, or a marketing mechanism for pharmaceutical companies. EBM, properly understood, should be a scientific tool for applying medical statistics to clinical practice. But using such a tool implies understanding both medical statistics and clinical practice, and having a medical, not an economic or political, goal.

17 Social and Economic Factors: Peer Review, Funding, and the Conventional Wisdom

Chapter 17

Science isn't a purely scientific process. As is now widely accepted – perhaps too accepted – many social and economic factors come into play. In this chapter, some of those factors will be reviewed, their impact will be explored, and common misinterpretations regarding those factors will be challenged.

Peer Review

The "best" scientific journals do not publish the most important articles. This viewpoint may be surprising but, if true, it will not be enough to read the largest and most famous journals. For new ideas, one must look elsewhere. The process of "peer review" is the major reason for this phenomenon.

The logistics of publishing scientific articles is a black box to most clinicians, and to the public. Unless one engages in research, one would not know all the human foibles that are involved. It is a quite fallible process, but one that seems to have some merit nonetheless.

The key feature is "peer review." The merits of peer review are debatable (Jefferson et al. 2002); indeed, its key feature of anonymity can bring out the worst of what has been called "the psychopathology of academe" (Mills 1963). Let us see how this works.

The process begins when the researcher sends an article to the editor of a scientific journal; the editor then chooses a few (usually 2–4) other researchers who usually are authorities in that topic; those persons are the peer reviewers and they are anonymous. The researcher does not know who they are. These persons then write 1–3 pages of review, detailing specific changes they would like to see in the manuscript. If the paper is not accurate, in their view, or has too many errors, or involves mistaken interpretations, and so on, the reviewers can recommend that it be rejected. The paper would then not be published by that journal, though the researcher could try to send it to a different journal and go through the same process. If the changes requested seem feasible to the editor, then the paper is sent back to the researcher with details of the changes requested by the peer reviewers. The researcher can then revise the manuscript and send it back to the editor; if all or most of the changes are made, the paper is then typically accepted for publication. Very rarely, reviewers may recommend acceptance of a paper with no or very minor changes from the beginning.

This is the process. It may seem rational, but the problem is that human beings are involved, and human beings are not, generally, rational. In fact, the whole scientific peer review process is, in my view, quite akin to Winston Churchill's definition of democracy: It is the worst system imaginable, except for all the others.

Perhaps the main problem is what one might call *academic road rage*. As is well known, it is thought that anonymity is a major factor that leads to road rage among drivers of automobiles. When I do not know who the other driver is, I tend to assume the worst about him; and when he cannot see my face, nor I his, I can afford to be socially inappropriate and aggressive, because facial and other physical cues do not impede me. I think the same factors are in play with scientific peer review: Routinely, one reads frustrated and angry comments from peer reviewers: exclamation points abound; inferences about one's intentions as an author are made based on pure speculation; one's integrity and research competence are not infrequently questioned. Now sometimes the content that leads to such exasperation is justifiable, and legitimate scientific and statistical questions can be raised – it is the emotion and tone which seem excessive.

Four Interpretations of Peer Review

Peer review has become a matter of explicit discussion among medical editors, especially in special issues of the *Journal of the American Medical Association* (*JAMA*). The result of this public debate has been summarized as follows:

> Four differing perceptions of the current refereeing process have been identified: "the sieve (peer review screens worthy from unworthy submissions), the switch (a persistent author can eventually get anything published, but peer review determines where, the smithy (papers are pounded into new and better shapes between the hammer of peer review and the anvil of editorial standards), and the shot in the dark (peer review is essentially unpredictable and unreproducible and hence, in effect, random)." It is remarkable that there is little more than opinion to support these characterizations of the gate-keeping process which plays such a critical role in the operation of today's huge medical research enterprise ("peer review is the linch pin of science"). (Silverman 1998, p. 27)

I tend to subscribe to the "switch" and "smithy" interpretations. I do not think that peer review is the wonderful sieve of the worthy from the unworthy that so many assume it to be, nor is it simply random. It is humanly irrational, however, and thus a troublesome "linchpin" for our science.

It is these human weaknesses that trouble me. For instance, peer reviewers often know authors, either personally or professionally, and they may have a personal dislike for an author; or they may dislike the author's ideas, in a visceral and emotional way. (Some even may have economic motivations, as some critics of the pharmaceutical industry suggest; see Healy 2001.) How can we remove these biases inherent in anonymous peer review? One approach would be to remove anonymity and force peer reviewers to identify themselves. Since all authors are peer reviewers for others, and all peer reviewers also write their own papers as authors, editors would be worried that they would not get complete and direct critiques from peer reviewers, who might fear retribution by authors (when serving as peer reviewers). Not just paper publication, but also grant funding – money, the life blood of a person's employment in medical research – are subject to anonymous peer review, and thus grudges that might be expressed in later peer review could in fact lead to losing funding and consequent economic hardship.

Who Reviews the Reviewers?

We see how far we have come from the neutral objective ideals of science. The scientific peer review process involves human beings of flesh and blood, who like and dislike each other, and the dollar bill, here as elsewhere, has a preeminent role.

How good or bad is this anonymous peer review process? I have described the matter qualitatively; are there any statistical studies of it? There are: one study, for example, decided to "review the reviewers" (Baxt et al. 1998). All reviewers of the *Annals of Emergency Medicine* received a fictitious manuscript, a purported placebo-controlled RCT of a treatment for migraine, for review in which 10 major and 13 minor statistical and scientific errors were deliberately placed. (Major errors included no definition of migraine, absence of any inclusion or exclusion criteria, and use of a rating scale that had never been validated or previously reported. Also, the p-values reported for the main outcome were made up and did not follow in any way from the actual data presented. The data demonstrated no difference between drug and placebo, but the authors concluded that there was a difference.) Of 203 reviewers, 15 recommend acceptance of the manuscript, 117 rejection, and 67 revision. So, about half of reviewers appropriately realized that the manuscript had numerous flaws, beyond the amount that would usually allow for appropriate revision. Further, 68% of reviewers did not realize that the conclusions written by the manuscript authors did not follow from other results of the study.

If this is the status of scientific peer review, then one has to be concerned that many studies are poorly vetted, and that some of the published literature is inaccurate either in its exposition, its interpretation, or in applying standard accepted statistical concepts.

Mediocrity Rewarded

Beyond the publication of papers that should not be published, the peer review process has the problem of not publishing papers that should be published. In my experience, both as an author and as an occasional guest editor for scientific journals, when multiple peer reviews bring up different concerns, it is impossible for authors to respond adequately to a wide range of critiques, and thus it is difficult for editors to publish. In such cases, the problem, perhaps, is not so much the content of the paper, but rather the topic itself. It may be too controversial, or too new, and thus difficult for several peer reviewers to agree that it merits publication.

In my own writing, I have noticed that, at times, the most rejected papers are the most enduring. My rule of thumb is that if a paper is rejected more than five times, then it is either completely useless or utterly prescient. In my view, scientific peer review ousts poor papers – but also great ones; the middling, comfortably predictable, ones tend to get published.

This brings us back to the claim made at the beginning of this chapter: that the most prestigious journals usually do not publish the most original or novel articles; this is because the peer review process is inherently conservative. I do not claim that there is any better system, but I think the weaknesses of our current system need to be honestly acknowledged.

One weakness is that scientific innovation is rarely welcomed, and new ideas are always at a disadvantage against the old and staid. Again, nonresearchers might have had a more favorable illusion about science – that it encourages progress and new ideas, and that it is consciously self-critical. That is how it should be; but this is how it is, again in the words of Ronald Fisher:

> A scientific career is peculiar in some ways. Its raison d'etre is the increase of natural knowledge. Occasionally, therefore, an increase of natural knowledge occurs. But this is tactless, and feelings are hurt. For in some small degree it is inevitable that views previously expounded are shown to be either obsolete or false. Most people, I think, can recognize this

and take it in good part if what they have been teaching for ten years or so comes to need a little revision; but some undoubtedly take it hard, as a blow to their amour proper, or even as an invasion of the territory they have come to think of as exclusively their own, and they must react with the same ferocity as we can see in the robins and chaffinches these spring days when they resent an intrusion into their little territories. I do not think anything can be done about it. It is inherent in the nature of our profession; but a young scientist may be warned and advised that when he has a jewel to offer for the enrichment of mankind some certainly will wish to turn and rend him. (Salsburg 2001a, p. 51)

So this is part of the politics of science – how papers get published. It is another aspect of statistics where we see numbers give way to human emotions, where scientific law is replaced by human arbitrariness. Even with all these limitations, we somehow manage to see a scientific literature that produces useful knowledge. The wise clinician will use that knowledge where possible, while remaining aware of the limitations of the process.

The Almighty Impact Factor

Many practitioners may not know that there is a private company, Thomson Reuters, owner of ISI (Information Sciences Institute), which calculates in a rather secretive fashion a quantitative score that drives much scientific research. This score, called the impact factor (IF), reflects how frequently papers are cited in the references of other papers. The more frequently papers are cited, presumably the more "impact" they are having on the world of research and practice. This calculation is relevant both for journals and for researchers. For journals, the more its articles are cited, the higher its impact factor and the greater its prestige, which, as with all things in our wonderfully capitalist world, translates into money: Advertisers and subscribers flock to the journals with the highest prestige, the greatest … impact. I participate in scientific journal editorial boards, and I have heard editors describe quite explicitly and calmly how they want to elicit more and more papers that are likely to have a high impact factor. Thus, given two papers that might be equally valid and solid scientifically, with one being on a "sexy" topic that generates much public interest, and another on a "nonsexy" topic, all other things being equal, the editor will lean toward the article that will interest readers more. Now this is not in itself open to criticism: we expect editors of popular magazines and newspapers to do the same. My point is that many clinicians and the public see science as such a stuffy affair that they may not realize that similar calculations go into the scientific publication process.

The impact factor also matters to individual researchers. Just as baseball players have batting averages by which their skills are judged, the IF is, in a way, a statistical batting average for medical researchers. In fact, ISI ranks researchers and produces a list of the ten most-cited scientific authors in each discipline. In psychiatry, for instance, the most cited author tends to be the first author of large epidemiological studies. Why is he cited so frequently? Because every time one writes a scientific article about depression, and begins with a generic statement like "Major depressive disorder is a common condition, afflicting 10% of the US population," that first author of the main epidemiologic studies of mental illness frequency is likely to be cited. Does such research move mountains? Not really. There is, no doubt, some relevance to the IF and some correlation with the value of scientific articles. There are data to back up this notion. Apparently, about 50% of scientific articles are never cited even once. The median rate of citation is only 1–2 citations; 50–100 citations would put an article above the 99th percentile, and more than 100 citations is the hallmark of a "classic" paper (Carroll 2006).

So IF captures something, but its correlation with quality research is not as strong or as direct as one might assume. One analysis looked at 131 articles publishing RCTs, and found that the quality of the studies was the same regardless of the impact factor (Barbui et al. 2006). Poorly cited studies were just as scientifically rigorous as highly cited ones.

So, IF must involve something more than research quality: this is where the politics of science is relevant. Topics that are in the public eye will have greater impact factors; researchers who are already well-established, and thus known to colleagues through conferences and personal contact, may have their work cited more frequently than unknown authors; and large research groups may inflate the IF scores of their colleagues by citing each other liberally in their publications. The rich get richer.

The Distorting Effect of the Impact Factor

One of my friends, currently a chairman of a department of psychiatry, described how his previous chair would sit down at Google Scholar and put in his name, and that of my friend, and whoever else was standing around, so as to compare the number of citations of the most popular papers each had published. In this way, scientific prestige, which used to be a more intuitively established matter, has become quantified. But the frequency with which people say one's name does not necessarily entail that one has much of importance to say.

The potential "distorting influence" of the IF on scientific research has begun to be recognized (Brown 2007). The decline in clinical research in medicine is especially relevant: clinical research is much less funded than basic animal research, and there are far fewer faculty members in medical schools who are clinical researchers as opposed to basic science researchers. Some think that this process is hastened because papers published by basic science researchers are more frequently cited by other scientists (and thus have a higher IF) than papers published by clinical researchers (Brown 2007). By judging faculty for promotion and retention based on the "impact" of their publications, medical schools would thus overestimate basic researchers and, conversely, underestimate the impact of clinical researchers. The IF is an imperfect and gross measure of the value of research, but "everyone loves a number" (Brown 2007).

The Intangibles of Coauthorship

Another aspect of the politics of science is self-censorship on the part of coauthors. Especially with large research papers (and perhaps more so if they are cowritten by employees or hires of the pharmaceutical industry), the interpretation of results tends to be driven in the favorable direction. This may be for various reasons: an obvious one is pecuniary interests when a study is pharmaceutically funded, but other, more intangible reasons may be just as important. Especially for large randomized clinical trials (RCTs), much money has been spent by someone (whether by taxpayers or pharmaceutical executives), and authors may feel the need to justify that expense. Further, such RCTs often take years to complete, and there are only so many years in a person's life; thus, authors may feel a need to think that they have been spending their lives wisely, producing important scientific results rather than failed data or debatable findings. The first authors tend to have spent more effort in such large studies than later authors, and thus they tend to drive the interpretive forces of published papers. In an interesting qualitative study (Horton 2002), a researcher found that 67% of contributors to research articles expressed reservations and concerns to him which they had not presented in the published paper. A certain amount of self-censorship seemed to be happening.

What Should We Believe?

Much has been made in recent years about the baneful influence of the pharmaceutical industry on medical research, and statistics, as enshrined in the evidence-based medicine movement (some call it "evidence-biased medicine"), is seen as an accomplice.

It is not new for statistics to be viewed with suspicion; as described previously, this was true long before the first pharmaceutical company ever existed. Indeed, it has long been known that statistics are prone to being misused: witness the famous comment by the nineteenth-century British prime minister Disraeli about lies, damn lies, and statistics.

This amenability to abuse is inherent in the nature of statistics; it can happen because using statistics is not just about the dry application of clear-cut rules, as many clinicians seem to assume. By now, in this book, this fact should be clear: statistics are chock full of assumptions and concepts and interpretations: in a word, numbers do not stand by themselves.

I hear clinicians say "I don't know who to believe anymore; so I won't believe anything." But it is not a matter of *belief*: it is a matter of science, properly conceived. It is not enough to say that we cannot take scientific studies at face value, and then to reject them all; we must learn how to *evaluate* them so that we know which ones to believe and which ones to discount.

Ghost Authorship

The first specter that we need to acknowledge is ghost authorship. This is the process whereby pharmaceutical companies draft scientific papers, later published under the "authorship" of academic researchers. I have seen this process from the inside. Usually, it occurs in the setting of a pharmaceutically designed multicenter clinical trial. The pharmaceutical company actually designs and writes the study protocol, often meant for FDA registration for a new drug. The company then recruits a number of academic and research sites to help conduct the study, get the patients who will enter it, and give the treatments and collect outcomes. The data that are produced are collected in a central site in the pharmaceutical company, analyzed by employee statisticians there. If the study shows no benefit, the process usually ends here. The results are never published (unpublished negative studies are discussed later), the drug is not taken to the FDA since it will be rejected, and the company turns to studying other drugs. If the results show that the drug is effective, then the company takes the data to the FDA for an official "indication" so that it can be marketed to the public. To publish the data in a scientific journal, the company often hires a medical writing company to prepare a first draft manuscript based on the data analysis by its statisticians. Then, researchers who were part of the study – those who had recruited patients for it and led its various research sites – are asked to be coauthors on the paper, and often they receive payments to be coauthors. They read the first draft manuscript, make suggestions for revision, and the company writers revise the paper accordingly. When submitted for publication in a scientific journal, the resulting paper does not usually have the name of any company employees or any individuals in the medical writing company. (Sometimes, in the middle or toward the end of the coauthor list, the company statistician and/or physician employees of the pharmaceutical company will be listed.) Usually, the first author and the following top authors are the most senior and recognized academic leaders among those who participated in designing and executing the study. Their role is often seen as legitimizing the study and lending the weight of their authority, as "key opinion leaders" (Moynihan 2008), to the results.

In the best conditions, I have observed, as a middle author among a list of 10 or more coauthors, that usually most of the comments regarding revision come from the first or second author and rarely from the other coauthors. And if the majority of authors make comments, they are usually quite minor. In effect, most coauthors are silent accomplices on the published paper. For them, this has the advantage of padding their resumes with one more paper, usually highly cited and published in prestigious journals (Patsopoulos, Ioannidis, and Analatos 2006). Thus, these resumes more quickly will appear to merit academic promotion to senior professorship positions. Critics of the pharmaceutical industry see – rightly, in my view – an unholy alliance where both sides benefit, at the cost of truth.

Who Has the Data?

One other factor is important: as described earlier, in almost all cases of large RCTs, the authors do not themselves analyze the data statistically; the analyses are conducted by company statisticians. When I have asked for access to the data myself, I am told that they are proprietary: private property, in effect, upon which I cannot trespass. Thus, unless the FDA requests them, scientists and the public can never confirm the actual data analyses themselves. One need not imagine actual data tampering, which would obviously be illegal, but, given our knowledge that statistics involve subjectivity, one can imagine analyses that are done and not reported, and analyses that are not reported exactly as they were done. For instance, an RCT may report a post-hoc positive result with a p-value of 0.01, but we have no denominator. We do not know if it was one positive result out of 5, or out of 335, analyses.

Unpublished Negative Studies

It is now well demonstrated that pharmaceutical industry sponsorship of studies correlates with positive results for the agent being studied (Lexchin et al. 2003), because negative studies tend to be unpublished. Since the first edition of this text, this problem has been solved to a great extent with the legal requirement that all studies be registered on a government website (www.clinicaltrials.gov), and that their results be made publicly available there, whether positive or negative, published or unpublished. This requirement is enforced by the US Food and Drug Administration (FDA), and noncompliance can lead to major penalties for pharmaceutical companies (such as restriction of drugs in the marketplace) or put at risk approval of important programs. Given these harms, pharmaceutical companies have been scrupulous about complying with this new regulation; academic researchers, who generally do not deal with the FDA, have not (DeVito and Goldacre 2021).

Clinical example: Antidepressant RCTs

This process has been best documented in a recent review of the FDA database of all 74 antidepressant clinical trials for unipolar depression in more than 12,000 subjects; 49% of studies were negative, and 51% were positive (Turner et al. 2008). Yet, since most negative studies were unpublished, the published literature was 94% positive (see Figure 17.1)

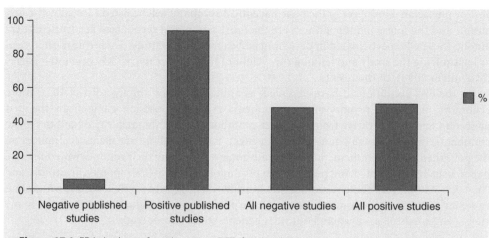

Figure 17.1 FDA database of antidepressant RCTs for unipolar depression: Comparison of studies published from that database and all studies in the database (including unpublished studies)

Further, of the negative studies, 61% were unpublished, 8% were published as frankly negative, but 31% were published as positive! This is usually where the negative primary outcomes are underplayed or even ignored, where the distinction between primary and secondary outcomes is not admitted, and where positive secondary outcomes are presented as if they were the main result of the study.

Unless a drug eventually receives FDA indication, a company is not required to provide all its data on that drug, including negative studies, to the FDA or anyone else. Thus, many drugs are simply ineffective, and proven so, but if they do not have an FDA indication for that condition, no one will know.

It is worth noting that a few exceptions exist where academic authors have published negative studies on a drug, but usually multiple negative RCTs are combined in one published paper (Pande et al. 2000; Kushner et al. 2006), producing much less impact than the usual multiple publications that ensue out of a single RCT (and usually found in the most read, most prestigious journals).

Clinical example: Lamotrigine in bipolar illness

In the past, the pharmaceutical industry did not make its negative data available routinely and fully on its websites; where such data was available, again as the result of litigation, important evidence of clinical inefficacy can be found (Ghaemi, Shirzadi, and Filkowski 2008). For instance, among the major companies with agents indicated for bipolar illness, only GlaxoSmithKline (GSK) provided data on its website regarding unpublished negative studies with results that were unfavorable to their product lamotrigine (Lamictal). Of nine studies provided at the GSK website, two were positive and published, and supported the company's success in securing an FDA-approved indication for lamotrigine for delay of relapse in the long-term treatment of bipolar illness patients (Calabrese et al. 2003; Bowden et al. 2003). Two negative studies have been published – one in rapid cycling (Calabrese et al. 2000) and another in acute bipolar depression (Calabrese et al. 1999) – but both published versions emphasize positive secondary outcomes as opposed to the negative primary outcomes. A negative study in rapid cycling has not been published in detail (GW611), nor have two negative randomized studies in acute bipolar depression (GW 40910 and GW 603), as well as two negative randomized trials in acute mania (GW609 and GW 610). A recent meta-analysis of five negative studies in acute bipolar depression is another example of the alchemy of turning dross to gold: when the five samples of about 200 patients each are pooled, the total sample of about 1,000 patients produces a positive p-value – but, not surprisingly, with a tiny effect size (about one point improvement on the Hamilton Depression Rating Scale) (Calabrese et al. 2008).

The clinical relevance of the lamotrigine studies is notable: Taking the negative outcomes into account, as of now, one might say that this agent is quite effective in maintenance treatment of bipolar illness, but it is not effective in acute mania, or rapid cycling, or perhaps acute bipolar depression. This context of where the drug is effective, and where it is not, is vital for scientifically valid and ethically honest clinical practice and research.

Disease-Mongering

Another aspect of clinical research that has come under scrutiny is the creation and expansion of diagnostic categories. Some critics argue that instead of discovering drugs for our diseases, we are creating diseases to match our drugs (Moynihan, Heath, and Henry 2002). This propensity seems most likely with single-symptom diagnoses, such as ADHD or social anxiety disorder. It has been claimed that even traditional diagnoses of centuries standing, such as bipolar disorder, may also be prone to it. Disease-mongering happens; many critics are so perturbed that they appear to suffer from the *disease of seeing disease-mongering everywhere*, and arguing that any increase in diagnosis of anything represents disease-mongering. Some diseases have been, and still are, underdiagnosed: bipolar disorder is one of them, AIDS is another. Increases in diagnoses of those conditions may reflect improved diagnostic practice.

Nonetheless, sometimes the marketing influence of pharmaceutically oriented research may not be directly about treatment studies, but rather about studies which promote increased diagnosis relevant to the treatment in question. Some have blamed the EBM movement for these practices, even though EBM concepts are not related to diagnostic studies. While I have not addressed specifics of diagnostic research in this book, it is relevant that some of these questionable marketing-oriented research practices can be critiqued by using Bayesian concepts, as in Chapter 13.

Follow the Money

Some critics have appeared to become proto-Marxists, insisting that the only factor that matters is economics. Follow the money, they say (Abramson 2004). If a doctor has any relationship with any pharmaceutical company funding, he must be biased; one author even advises patients to fire their doctors on this basis alone (Angell 2005). This kind of postmodernist criticism – seeing nothing but power and money as the source of all knowledge – seems simplistic, to say the least (Dennett 2000). Even government funding can be related to bias. It may be in fact that the bias has less to do with funding than with researchers' own belief-systems, their ideologies (another concept derivable from Karl Marx). This is a complex topic, but a source of evidence that argues against an economic reductionist model is that about one-quarter of all psychiatric research is not even funded at all, *by any source* (Silberman and Snyderman 1997). Often, those unfunded studies are sources of important new ideas.

Avoiding Nihilism

These critiques are not meant to engender a nihilistic reaction in the reader. It is not necessary to think nothing is meaningful simply because science is complex. Having read this far, readers should not conclude that the scientific literature is useless. They should, I hope, use this book to be able to navigate the scientific literature. There are more than enough voices on the internet and elsewhere of those who take a one-sided view: everything is horrible, or everything is perfect. The truth is never so simple.

Thinking back to the first section of this book, where I highlighted that all facts are theory-laden, it may also be relevant to point out that the influence of bias in clinical research is not limited to the pharmaceutical industry. Even government-funded studies can be biased for the simple reason that although money is influential, human beings are also motivated by other desires: Perhaps chief among these is prestige, which from Plato to Hegel has been recognized as perhaps the ultimate human desire. Many researchers, subtly or obviously, consciously or unconsciously, are biased by their wish to be right. Sometimes the truth takes a back seat when defending one's opinions. It is quite difficult for any person to be fully free of this hubris. Sometimes, it completely takes over and destroys one. A sobering example, useful to show how influences other than money can matter, is a prominent case of a PhD researcher who specialized in diabetes research. For a decade he obtained numerous NIMH grants which led to much prestige. His research was not unusual; in fact, he apparently doctored his data so that his results would agree with the academic mainstream, thus ensuring him more governmental funding and academic prestige (Sox and Rennie 2006). He went to prison.

Researcher bias can, and does, occur for many reasons. While efforts are needed to clean up academic medicine, clinicians will always need to hone and use their ultimate tool: knowledge.

18 The New Canon of Psychopharmacology (STAR*D, STEP-BD, CATIE): How Clinical Trials Are Misinterpreted

In the mid-1990s, an incredible thing happened: The NIMH decided to fund major clinical psychopharmacology studies. About 90% of NIMH is for other purposes, so the world of clinical psychopharmacology always has suffered from neglect in academic research. The field has relied on the pharmaceutical industry for its largest and most definitive studies, with all the limitations already discussed. NIMH leadership, almost always laboratory researchers without background in clinical psychopharmacology, has tended to see this problem as a solution. Government funding wasn't needed where private industry funding was present.

By now it should be obvious how harmful this attitude has been.

Besides the scientific reasons for government funding of psychopharmacology research, the mid-1990s provided an opportunity in the United States for the first and only time in the past half century. For a few brief golden years, the federal government under the Clinton administration had a budget surplus. The NIMH had extra money, and it decided to spend a little more, finally, on clinical psychopharmacology.

Those budgets may have seemed large to academic researchers, but they weren't huge: about $20 million each for the three studies funded in the three major psychiatric diseases of severe depression, bipolar illness, and schizophrenia. Much has been made of these studies, and they will be discussed in detail here, but it is relevant to note that $20 million is tiny in the world of pharmaceutical research. That amount would be spent on a few Phase II trials, with about 100 subjects or so, just to get to the point of deciding whether to do much larger Phase III trials for marketing approval. Those Phase III trials tend to run in the hundreds of millions of dollars in psychiatry for each drug. So, $20 million to study most available major drugs for a major illness is not much.

But these few drops of water felt wonderful to the parched throats of the field of government-funded clinical psychopharmacology.

Of course, the federal budget quickly fell into debt and has remained there for the past three decades. These studies will not be repeated and, with all their limitations, they are and will remain for the near future the best data available on clinical psychopharmacology with current agents outside of pharmaceutical industry studies.

These studies thus have been called the "canons of psychiatry" when used for teaching in a family medicine setting (Brazill, Warnick, and White 2018); they are a canon, but one that has been misread.

The New Canon of Psychopharmacology

So, what is this new canon of psychiatry – or, more properly, the new canon of psychopharmacology?

We have three studies: for schizophrenia, the Clinical Antipsychotic Trials of Intervention Effectiveness (CATIE); for so-called major depressive disorder, the Sequenced Treatment Alternatives to Relieve Depression (STAR*D); and for bipolar illness, the Systemic Treatment Enhancement Program for Bipolar Disorder (STEP-BD). These grants were contracts given to consortia of universities: $20 million or so would be spread about between 10 or so universities. The universities would be sites in a single trial, designed by a core site. CATIE was headed by and centrally designed out of Columbia University, while STAR*D and STEP-BD were headed by and centrally designed out of Massachusetts General Hospital (MGH)/Harvard Medical School. I participated in some of the early work on STEP-BD at MGH, and later headed a subsite of that study at Cambridge Hospital/Harvard Medical School, so I observed some of the sausage-making process, as well as the later presentation of results.

Most of the research was conducted in the early 2000s and then published later in that decade and into the 2010s. Hundreds of papers have been produced, and careers have been made and advanced with this work.

Let's review how the studies mainly have been interpreted and presented, and then look at alternative interpretations of those studies, focusing on the statistical methods that will adjudicate what are the most correct interpretations.

The Main Rationale for These Studies

There are some common rationales for these three studies. The first is that pharmaceutical industry funding tends to take a cookbook approach to satisfy regulatory standards (from the Food and Drug Administration [FDA] in the United States) to come to the commercial market. These standards require that each drug be shown to be more effective than placebo in two separate trials. In American psychiatry, there generally is no FDA requirement that a drug be shown to be equal or better than prior proven treatments. Hence, we have hundreds of studies comparing single antidepressants or antipsychotics versus placebo, as reviewed previously. But we have very few studies directly comparing individual antidepressants or antipsychotics to each other. "Network" meta-analysis is a false solution to this problem.

Hence, clinicians in practice do not know if one drug is better than another, or what they should do if one drug fails. They basically have to guess.

These studies had a general principle of trying to help clinicians answer those questions. Thus, the CATIE and STAR*D didn't have placebo arms since efficacy of individual drugs over placebo was considered proven already. Instead, they were designed mainly to compare each drug to another.

A related rationale for conducting these studies was to address the concern that pharmaceutical-industry-conducted or -sponsored studies tend to be biased in favor of the drug being studied. For those who harbor doubts regarding the biasing effects of the pharmaceutical industry, the conduct of studies by academic groups without commercial consequences, funded by the federal government, would seem to make it more likely that results would be less biased in favor of drugs.

A final comment is that STEP-BD differed from CATIE and STAR*D in including a placebo arm. Unlike the immense literature in schizophrenia and depressive illness, the bipolar literature on antidepressants was sparse. Hence, STEP-BD had much more modest goals than CATIE or STAR*D; it simply wanted to see if antidepressants were better than placebo. Despite its simple design, even STEP-BD has been misinterpreted in practice.

The Conventional Wisdom: CATIE for Schizophrenia

Here is the official line on the design and results of these studies: CATIE was a one year study of schizophrenia, in which a large sample of about 1,500 patients were recruited at about 50 clinical trial sites (exact numbers are n = 1,493 in 57 sites). They were randomized double-blind to one of five drugs: olanzapine, risperidone, quetiapine, ziprasidone, and perphenazine. The first four agents were second-generation dopamine blockers, and the last agent was a first-generation traditional dopamine blocker. There was no placebo arm.

The basic question was whether second-generation dopamine blockers are more effective than a first-generation dopamine blocker in long-term treatment of schizophrenia. Secondary questions were whether the second-generation agents were more tolerable than the first, and whether any differences within second-generation agents could be seen on effectiveness and tolerability.

The commonly cited interpretation of the results is simple:

All antipsychotics were similar in efficacy and tolerability. End of story.

Alternative Interpretation: Effectiveness – What Is the Outcome Being Measured?

What this simple interpretation overlooks is that they were similarly ineffective, or hardly effective. The main outcome was discontinuation of medication at one year. That's a very low standard; it doesn't involve improvement in schizophrenia symptom scores, much less functional improvement, which would be the real test of long-term effectiveness in schizophrenia. But simply asking the question "Do patients stay on their drugs and do doctors keep patients on those drugs for up to one year?", the answer was "No" in about three-quarters of patients (range 64–82%, depending on the drug). Since there was no placebo, we can't know if the quarter or so who remained on their antipsychotic would have benefited more than if they had received nothing/placebo. But when three-quarters of patients do poorly with a treatment, a question would seem to arise as to whether that treatment is effective.

Again, it can be argued that those treatments already are proven effective, but those studies were pharmaceutical industry-sponsored trials for market approval, which are 3 month studies for acute exacerbation benefit using schizophrenia symptom rating scales.

In other words, the outcomes were different. The studies which allow antipsychotics to be on the general market show benefit over three months for acute worsening of symptoms. The CATIE trial tried to test a modest measure of longer-term benefit – drug discontinuation up to one year – and it found that most patients did not benefit with antipsychotic treatment of any kind. It could be argued, of course, that there are maintenance studies of antipsychotics that show benefit over placebo for up to one year of treatment, but those studies look at different outcomes than CATIE; also, most commonly relapse into an acute exacerbation (Goff et al. 2017). They do not show improvement in chronic psychosis over time.

Hence, in contrast to the planned comparison of one drug versus another drug, the CATIE trial only answers that question by raising more questions about how effective these drugs are.

The researchers who conducted the study have emphasized that this alternative interpretation should not be taken, but it seems not unreasonable given the lower overall effectiveness rates in the study.

The methodological take-home point is that you can't change your outcomes when you're comparing to the literature. CATIE assumed that the outcomes of 3 month trials would extend to a year and allow drug-versus-drug comparisons. The outcomes at a year were poor enough, though, to throw into doubt any efficacy at all.

Alternative Interpretation: Tolerability – Forget P-Values

The other major conventional wisdom interpretation of CATIE was that most drugs had similar tolerability, and specifically that the older antipsychotic perphenazine was similar in its extrapyramidal side effects to the modern antipsychotics.

This matter has been described in more detail in Chapter 7 where it was shown that this false equivalence was based on a standard mistake: the misuse of p-values. CATIE was not powered statistically to show differences in the lower absolute frequencies seen with extrapyramidal side effects (EPS). Hence, a false negative error is present. Using confidence intervals, differences can be shown to exist (with an irrelevance of the concept of statistical significance), such as lower overall EPS rates with quetiapine compared to other agents.

The Conventional Wisdom: STAR*D for Depression

The second large canon of psychopharmacology is the STAR*D study, a large sequential randomized clinical trial (RCT) of more than 1,000 patients with an acute depressive episode of so-called major depressive disorder (Rush et al. 2006). Before STAR*D, there were few RCTs comparing antidepressants to each other, and hardly any looking at outcomes after multiple failed trials.

The main outcome was to assess whether there was a difference between switching antidepressants versus combining them as adjuncts, after failure of initial antidepressant monotherapy.

The STAR*D protocol was as follows: First, 1,439 patients were treated openly with citalopram. If they failed to respond (n = 727), they were then randomized double-blind to a different monoamine agonist or combination with two monoamine agonists (or other adjunctive agents like buspirone). If they failed this second trial, they were randomized to switching to tricyclic antidepressants (TCAs) or augmentation with lithium or thyroid hormone. If they failed this third trial, they were randomized to a monoamine oxidase inhibitor or the combination of venlfaxine plus mirtazapine.

Response rates are shown in Figure 18.1.

The standard interpretation put forward by the researchers who conducted STAR*D was that there was no difference between switching versus combining antidepressants for refractory depression. A secondary conclusion was that most patients (about 2/3) improved after multiple antidepressant trials for an acute depressive episode (Rush et al. 2006a).

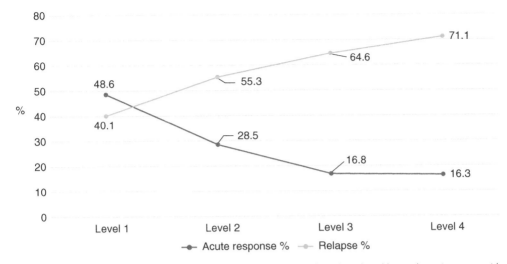

Figure 18.1 STAR*D: Acute response declines by half of subjects with each trial, and later relapse increases with each trial to over half of subjects

Alternative Interpretations of STAR*D

The main outcome seems straightforward. Combining antidepressants versus switching agents did not differ notably. Thus, the primary outcome of STAR*D was not too controversial. The result would argue for switching antidepressants after initial nonresponse, since fewer side effects should ensue with one versus more agents.

Alternative interpretations become relevant to the secondary claim that most patients eventually improve. A closer look at the data finds that this 2/3 full interpretation is really only 2/3 empty.

As can be seen in Figure 18.1, treatment response was good in the first two episodes, but fell by half thereafter. By the fourth monoamine agonist trial, only 15% of subjects respond to any new treatments, even the most potent agents known: the MAOIs.

Besides the acute response issue, it is important to note that patients continued to be followed for up to a year, so that continuation of response was able to be assessed. On that outcome, it was found that even if patients responded, about 40–70% relapsed within one year even if they stayed on the same agents which had led to acute response.

So the 2/3 initial response has to be cut by half for continued response, which leads to about 1/3 response up to one year. Again, the absence of a placebo group raises the question of whether this response would be higher than natural history.

Further, the addition of response by treatment trial after trial obscures the fact that acute response fell markedly by the third trial, so that after that point, further agents had a very low likelihood of acute treatment response (only about 15%). That's not good news. If a patient sees a clinician in a current depression that has failed to respond to 2–3 prior agents, the clinician would, based on STAR*D, have to tell the patient that there is a 85% likelihood of not getting better no matter what other antidepressants are used, including MAOIs.

STAR*D addressed one point well: that of switch rather than augment antidepressants for refractory depression. But it raised other questions: First, like CATIE, are antidepressants long-term at all? Second, does anything work after a few failed trials?

The methodological take-home point is that even in a well-conducted clinical trial in which the primary objective is answered, like STAR*D, the secondary results can be very important clinically. And those results should not be interpreted in the most positive way possible alone, as done by the STAR*D researchers, but with attention to the maximum information one can derive from them. STAR*D tells us that antidepressant benefit declines over time, from 2/3 initially to 1/3 later, and that antidepressant benefit declines markedly after a few initial failed trials. These are important conclusions, though they tend to be ignored because they show that antidepressants are much less effective than is commonly presumed.

The Conventional Wisdom: STEP-BD for Bipolar Depression

CATIE was the largest (about 1,500 patients) and most ambitious of the three canons of psychopharmacology; it failed to show that most patients even stay on their medications for a year in schizophrenia. STAR*D was about half the size of CATIE (around 750 patients), but still large, and showed benefit acutely, but, again, most patients did not stay well with their medications for a year with depression. STEP*BD was smaller again, about half the size of STAR*D, but very different in its goals. The efficacy of lithium and other mood stabilizers for long-term treatment was well-established. What was controversial was short-term treatment, specifically with antidepressants.

Thus, a 6-month acute trial of 366 patients was designed comparing bupropion versus paroxetine versus placebo for acute bipolar depression (Sachs et al. 2007). Both of those agents had been studied previously and found to have low mania switch rates, which is why they were chosen. The result of the main study was that both agents were equivalent to placebo.

The simple conclusion was that antidepressants were proven equal to placebo and thus ineffective in bipolar depression. A secondary outcome was that mania switch rates also were equal in all three arms, and thus these antidepressants were shown not to cause mania any more than placebo.

In short, antidepressants didn't help, but they also didn't hurt. Since most clinicians used antidepressants in most patients with bipolar illness, the researchers didn't argue against that practice; in fact antidepressant use in bipolar illness has not declined, and has actually increased somewhat since STEP-BD was published.

Alternative Interpretations of STEP-BD: Bayesian Aspects

The main result of STEP-BD would seem very straightforward. When a drug is equivalent to placebo, the standard interpretation is that the drug doesn't work, assuming adequate statistical power and other clinical trial methods, which was the case in STEP-BD. But it's one thing to say that a drug doesn't work before it comes to the commercial market, as is the case before FDA indications. When drug companies have results of a new medication that are equivalent to placebo, they won't even bother taking it to the FDA. They know it will be rejected. If a drug isn't being used, then equivalence to placebo means it won't be used.

But what happens when a drug already is in use, and commonly so, as with antidepressants in bipolar depression? Despite absence of FDA indication for that purpose, antidepressants are on the commercial market for other depressive conditions, and clinicians believe they work for bipolar depression also. The STEP-BD results arrive, therefore, in a context that is quite different than when a drug is being developed by a pharmaceutical company before it is taken to the FDA to possibly enter the market. The issue now with antidepressants in bipolar depression is that the results of STEP-BD, showing inefficacy, would have to convince clinicians *to stop* using those agents, as opposed to not letting them do so at all. This is a very different scenario.

The situation can be understood through the lens of the preceding chapter: Bayesian statistics. The same study result can mean very different things in different settings. Where no one knows anything about a drug, a study showing placebo equivalence would mean that no one would believe in it. When people already believe in a drug, a study showing placebo equivalence might influence some fence-straddlers, but for the majority who strongly believe in drug efficacy, reasons will be found to keep doing what they're doing.

In the case of antidepressants in bipolar depression, the reason was the second outcome: the drugs didn't cause acute manic switch more than placebo. So, if they don't hurt, and if I believe they work, I'll keep using them, reasoned many a clinician.

A Bayesian analysis could get into the other harmful effects of antidepressants not measured in STEP-BD, such as their long-term mood-destabilizing effects causing rapid cycling in about 1/4 of patients. But the STEP-BD researchers did not address those issues, and many clinicians came away with a Bayesian interpretation which they didn't realize was Bayesian: they allowed a partial assessment of the scientific literature, excluding other known harms, to allow them to downplay the implications of the inefficacy shown with antidepressants in STEP-BD.

The methodological take-home point is that Bayesian analysis can be distorted if it isn't as complete and objective as possible.

Alternative Interpretations of STEP-BD: Concomitant Medications

As with CATIE, we see a misuse of p-values in STEP-BD's analysis of acute manic switch, to claim a false equivalence between drugs and placebo. STEP-BD was not powered to assess whether bupropion or placebo cause manic switch. Thus, the absence of a statistical difference cannot be claimed to show no difference. Again, p-values are misused and effect sizes and confidence intervals should have been used, as shown previously with CATIE. Of the antidepressant group, 10.1% (18/179) had manic switch, versus 10.7% (20/187) of the placebo group. In this case the direction of effect, if any, is slightly in the direction of placebo. Of course, there is no biological or clinical rationale for antidepressants reducing the risk of manic switch, so this result likely is not meaningful. More importantly, both groups were also taking baseline mood stabilizers, which reduce the risk of manic switch. Thus, the key factor here may not be that misuse of p-values obscured a real effect, but the effect of concomitant medications, namely treatment with anti-manic agents, that may have prevented the observation of any potential risk.

An analogy would be as follows: Suppose you were doing a study of a drug which might cause fever, but all patients were treated with anti-fever drugs like aspirin at the same time. If that drug had similar fever rates as placebo, in patients treated with anti-fever treatment with aspirin, would you then conclude that the drug inherently doesn't cause fever?

Summary of the Canon of Psychopharmacology

So, what does the canon of psychopharmacology teach us? An important lesson is that even though the studies were conducted outside the realm of the pharmaceutical industry, by academic centers and with government funding, in each case the researchers seemed strongly biased toward the most positive favorable spin they could give to the drugs being studied. This result stands out especially because the studies found, each in its own way, that the drugs being studied were less effective than had been presumed before these studies were conducted. Many of the more complex questions the studies were designed to answer, such as relative efficacy between agents, could not even be addressed because of the overall low effectiveness of the medications for these illnesses.

Methodologically, the main way in which researchers gave their most positive spin to these studies was by Bayesian interpretations where the weak results of these specific studies were downplayed in the context of partial and positively biased interpretations of the scientific literature. Besides that aspect, researchers also interpreted secondary results in a positive and partial manner, such as ignoring relapse after acute recovery in commonly cited STAR*D figures or ignoring false negative results due to misuse of p-values in CATIE and STEP-BD tolerability outcomes.

How to Analyze a Study

Much of this book is intended to provide readers the tools to analyze research studies which they read or hear about in scientific journals. A recent US Veterans Administration (VA) study on lithium (Katz et al. 2022) provides a good example of why it is important to analyze research studies for yourself. Don't rely on what the authors tell you, and don't rely on the journal reviewers to vet the study sufficiently.

This recent study reported that lithium did not differ from placebo in prevention of suicide-related outcomes over 1 year in 519 patients. The study was stopped early due to this lack of difference in interim analysis. The authors are to be commended for making the effort to conduct such an important and difficult study. Their extensive efforts in data collection deserve the highest quality of data analysis and scientific interpretation.

If the study had positive results, it would have been surprising, but definitive. Lithium would have been proven effective in reducing all kinds of suicidality – fatal, nonfatal, serious, mild, attempts, ideas – in all kinds of patients – bipolar, unipolar, substance abuse, PTSD. The study did not have that result. But a negative result does not mean the opposite, namely that lithium has no anti-suicidal effect at all, not only because of a larger scientific literature proving otherwise, but also because of some of this study's own results.

What the paper did not describe is a simple observation: there were two groups in the study – those with bipolar illness and those with "major depression." The study reported the outcomes in each group separately but it didn't analyze those outcomes, which, had they been analyzed, would have shown likely benefit in the bipolar subgroup.

So, let's review how the study should have been analyzed, beginning with a general approach to take to all studies, whether they report positive results, or negative ones, as in this case.

How to Approach Any Paper

The key is to look at all the tables and figures. Forget about the abstract and introduction. Don't even read them. Come back to the methods later, after seeing the results. Go straight to the results, and don't bother with the text. Start with the tables and figures.

There are two basic types of content to tables and figures: predictors and outcomes. Predictors are the baseline characteristics of the sample. Outcomes are the endpoints of the study.

The whole point of randomization is to equalize predictors, and most studies of sufficient size do so. Sometimes studies have inclusion criteria that will bias the result based on predictors. For instance, the drug group may be naïve, never treated before with the drug, while a comparison group might include nonresponders to a standard comparison. The methods section should be assessed to look for such difference between groups before it even begins.

Outcomes reflect the effects of treatment, either with drug or placebo. If randomization was successful and predictors are similar in both groups, then outcome differences can be interpreted as causal.

Application to This Study

Let's apply these principles to this study:

Let's go to the tables and figures: First there is table 1, the baseline demographic and clinical characteristics of the sample. There were little differences there. There were more "other mental disorders" in the lithium group (30% vs 19% for placebo), but it was not clear what those conditions were, and I let it slide.

Table 19.1 Patient outcomes by treatment and psychiatric diagnosis (originally Table 2 in the cited paper)

Characteristic	n	Lithium n(%)	Placebo n(%)
n		255	264
First and subsequent suicide attempts	197	96 (49%)	101 (51%)
Bipolar disorder	30	10 (33%)	20 (67%)
MDD	167	86 (51%)	81 (49%)

Adapted from Katz et al 2022. Partial presentation of full table. MDD = major depressive disorder. Note that 1/3 of all cases of suicide attempts in bipolar illness happened in lithium-treated patients versus 2/3 of all suicide attempts cases in bipolar illness happening in placebo-treated patients. Applying relative risk (RR) estimates and confidence intervals (CI), RR = 2.0 with 95% CIs of 1.1, 3.5, which does not include the null value and thus is statistically meaningful. One could also look at the outcomes as in the text, dividing by the denominator of overall subjects with bipolar illness in the study (n=80), again finding about twice as much suicide attempts in the placebo group versus the lithium group. No difference existed for MDD. Percentages for the lower two rows were added here; they are not found in the original paper.

Next was table 2, which reflects patient outcomes. The first line was "Primary outcomes, first and subsequent events" and it was immediately divided into "bipolar illness" and "major depressive disorder" (MDD).

Scanning table 2, the bipolar and MDD groups are equal or similar on all outcomes down the line, except for the very first line for bipolar disorder, where there is a clear difference: 10 cases for lithium and 20 cases for placebo. That's a two-fold difference, which is a major effect. There was no notable difference for major depressive disorder. From there, the reader simply can go to the methods to see how many patients with bipolar illness were included in the study. There were 80 patients, distributed as 37 for lithium and 43 for placebo. That is a small percentage (15%) of the overall sample of more than 500 subjects, but the effect size is so large – a doubling of effect – that it was worth making an analysis to see if this difference was statistically significant despite the small subgroup size.

The subgroup thus consisted of 10/37 lithium patients versus 20/43 placebo patients who had the primary outcomes in first and subsequent events. You could simply divide these numbers and get numbers of 27% for lithium vs 46.5% for placebo. The eyeballs already saw the doubling of effect with placebo over lithium; the percentages give exact numbers. All that is left is to get confidence intervals and p-values to establish statistical significance. Standard statistical software allows one to insert the raw numbers in a 2 × 2 table for the two groups, and the software applies the standard equations for confidence intervals to provide a relative risk and 95% confidence intervals.

A simple analysis of the raw data from the paper demonstrates that the relative risk of a suicidal outcome on placebo was about twice as high as with lithium (RR = 1.72) with 95% confidence intervals that include the null value, meaning that the result is technically not statistically significant, but which skews strongly in the direction of more benefit with lithium (lower CI 0.93, upper CI 3.20).

Other Tables and Figures

One could go on and look at other tables and figures. Figure 2 was the primary outcome of all suicidal phenomena, showing no difference between groups, but the subgroup effect of bipolar illness would not be visible in that figure. Table 3 had hazard ratios for outcomes with models using different predictors, including different types of suicidal phenomena. In that table, we could talk further about the authors' inappropriate exclusion of three suicides with placebo in their analysis, although they included one suicide with lithium, but for now we will leave that question aside.

In general, in table 3, the authors tried to look at different predictors and subgroups and they kept finding no differences. But they never bothered to look at the bipolar subgroup. Why? The difference was obvious and leaped out in the first row of table 2, but there is no comment about this difference anywhere in the text.

As noted, the study reported the outcomes in each group separately but it didn't analyze those outcomes. When one does so, there is clear statistically significant benefit in the bipolar subgroup. Why did the authors not do this analysis? Why did the peer reviewers not ask for it?

It's important to note that most clinical researchers in psychiatry are not trained formally in statistics, such as with a public health biostatistics degree. Unfortunately, neither the main authors nor the reviewers usually have the statistical expertise to notice such an issue. Authors tend to rely on a statistician for their study, but statisticians do not have the clinical knowledge base to identify important issues of concern. Things easily fall between the cracks.

As a reader of the scientific literature, you have to fill the cracks. Don't read the text. Study the tables and figures, and do your own analyses. Then you will either confirm the authors' findings, or you might reinterpret the study more accurately than the authors themselves have done.

Critiques

One might claim that this subgroup analysis has a high false-positive possibility, since it was not a primary outcome and it is one of many possible comparisons. However, this group is exactly the group where lithium's benefits have been shown most clearly for half a century. Hence, this is not a random subgroup analysis, like an astrological sign, but one founded on a huge scientific evidence base that is consistent with the observed result.

Thus, one interpretation of the study is that lithium does reduce suicidal activity in bipolar illness, but perhaps not in nonbipolar illness.

Even that conclusion might be too strong, though, because it is important to distinguish suicide attempts from parasuicidal behavior. Suicide attempts are acts with intent to die, such as hanging or overdose. Parasuicidal behavior reflects self-harm without intent to die and with nonfatal means, such as self-cutting or cigarette burning on the skin. It would have been helpful if the study differentiated suicide attempts from parasuicidal behavior, but the published paper does not do so. The main meta-analysis upon which the causal relationship between lithium use and suicide prevention is based made this distinction: lithium was effective in prevention of completed suicide; it was not effective in reduction of parasuicidal behavior. Since parasuicidal behavior reflects at least part of the outcomes in this study, the result is consistent with the main prior meta-analysis that showed lithium prevents completed suicide but does not benefit parasuicidal behavior. The present study does not address, much less refute, the prior meta-analysis of randomized studies that lithium prevents completed suicide.

Data Buried in the Text

The key issue of completed suicide is a good example of how relevant data, not definitive yet still important, can be buried in the text of a study.

Completed suicide could not be addressed definitively by this study because, thankfully, such outcomes are rare. This is why randomized trials of suicidality really aren't studies of suicide, but studies of suicide attempts or ideation, which is not the same thing. Nonetheless, it is important to note that here also, in completed suicide, this study showed a benefit with lithium.

There were four completed suicides in or around the study: one with lithium and three with placebo. This result is a three-fold elevated risk with placebo over lithium. The study authors stated that the numbers were too few to calculate a difference. That's not the case. Differences always can be calculated; whether they are meaningful or not is another question. Of course, with these small numbers 95% statistical significance is not achievable, but that does not mean the results are meaningless. A 2×2 table analysis provides a relative risk of 2.92, with 95% lower and upper confidence intervals of 0.30 and 27.8. This means that the confidence with which one would see this result ranges from a 70% possibility of increased risk with lithium and an equally likely possibility of a 27-fold (or 2,700%) probability of increased risk with lithium. Since the null value is one, these confidence intervals are highly skewed in the direction of more harm with placebo and protection with lithium. Of course, one could argue that the results are so few that one more case of completed suicide in the lithium arm would make the two groups equal. That is the case, but the possibility that this result is real should be considered given that four prior randomized trials found benefit with lithium in prevention of completed suicide, as meta-analyzed previously.

Scientific research does not happen in a vacuum. No single study is definitive. As taught in the Bayesian approach, one should interpret a new study in the context of prior knowledge, so as to revise one's perspective based on that knowledge. Taking an all-or-nothing approach ("it works or it doesn't work") is not productive since it ignores the total literature.

It should be noted that lithium has been shown to prevent completed suicide in randomized clinical trials. This study is consistent with those results, not contradictory. Also, there is a large geological literature which finds much higher suicide rates in populations where lithium levels in the ground are near-absent. These data imply that very low lithium doses, equivalent to about 25 mg/d of lithium carbonate, could prevent suicide. Again, this study, which had subtherapeutic levels for mood illness but high levels compared to the geological studies, does not refute that literature because it too found lower completed suicide rates with lithium than with placebo.

In sum: Lithium has been shown to prevent suicide attempts in bipolar illness; this study has the same finding, not a contradictory result. The nonbipolar population in this study is heterogenous, not simply "unipolar" depressive, including a high substance abuse rate, so the lack of benefit with lithium in that group is difficult to interpret. However, lithium has been found not to be effective in reducing parasuicidal behavior, which tends to occur in populations without severe mood illness. This study is consistent with that literature, not contradictory to it.

This study has been misreported as somehow contradicting the prior lithium literature. Instead, it confirms it: There is lack of benefit for parasuicidal behavior in general, but there is benefit for suicide attempts in bipolar illness, and there is numerical benefit for completed suicide. Unfortunately, the study authors did not analyze differences when seen, such as the statistically significant benefit for prevention of suicide attempts in the bipolar illness subgroup. And the study did not attempt to understand the relevance of completed suicide, as opposed to other suicidal behavior, where, with the few completed suicides that occurred, the results again did not contradict the prior literature showing lithium benefit.

Methodological Conclusions

No single study is definitive, and every RCT should be used to help plan better ones.

This study should be used to learn important lessons to further clarify the evidence base regarding lithium and suicide. Randomized studies in suicidality are extremely difficult to do. Completed suicide is infrequent, and thus it is impossible to do a large enough study for a long enough time to adequately power a primary outcome of completed suicide. Such a study likely would be unethical in any case. So suicidality studies tend to use composite outcomes: suicide attempts with fatal intent, suicide attempts without fatal intent, suicide attempts with potentially fatal methods, suicide attempts without potentially fatal methods, parasuicidal self-harm, increase in suicidal ideation, new suicidal ideation – all these aspects of suicidality are combined in one composite outcome, along with the rare outcome of completed suicide. This mixing of suicidal ideas and behaviors in one outcome is understandable statistically; a higher frequency of an outcome is obtained, thereby reducing the sample size needed for statistical power. However, it comes at a cost: the outcome is noisy, and one outcome could go in one direction while another goes in the opposite direction, producing an average with no change. This possibility is the case especially with the general difference between suicide attempts or intent with potentially fatal methods, and self-harm of a nonfatal nature. This study confirms the prior literature that these two aspects of suicidality should be separated.

Future randomized studies of this topic should focus on excluding parasuicidal behavior, such as self-cutting. Only suicide attempts that are fatal in intent or method should be included. Further, future randomized studies should be conducted only in bipolar illness, in one set of studies, and only in nonbipolar illness, in other sets of studies, so that the different patient populations can be effectively analyzed. Lastly, completed suicide is not amenable to randomized research, and no single study can address that topic. All future randomized research on lithium should be seen as relevant to noncompleted suicidal behavior only. The completed suicide literature will remain as it is, showing benefit with lithium, until future meta-analyses can aggregate sufficient outcomes to update the current evidence base.

Summary

This chapter provides a good example of how to approach reading a clinical trial study article. Key points are the following:

> Never take the results simply at face value from the abstract.
> Don't rely on the abstract at all.
> Always look at the tables and figures. They'll provide most of the story.
> Look in the text for important buried data.
> No study is definitive; always interpret it in a Bayesian manner in
>   relation to the entire literature.

With a complex topic like suicide, use the results of an RCT with complex results, such as this one, to design better trials to test possible benefit more cleanly.

False Positive Maintenance Clinical Trials in Psychiatry

Although classical randomized clinical trials (RCTs) are the gold standard for proof of drug efficacy, the Food and Drug Administration (FDA) has increasingly allowed a different design, called randomized discontinuation trials (RDTs), for indication purposes (FDA 2019). These RDTs, called "enriched," are used routinely in psychiatric maintenance trials for FDA registration. This chapter examines the benefits and limitations of RDTs, and concludes that their extensive use in psychiatric maintenance studies may compromise scientific validity. The core critique here is with the *concept* of RDTs – that is, their internal validity, not just their external validity or misuse or misinterpretation.

Rationale for the RDT Design

The enriched RDT design involves the following scenario: To prove long-term maintenance efficacy of a psychiatric drug, patients who enter a double-blind RCT are initially selected, before the study begins, to receive the relevant medication nonrandomly for an acute phase of the illness (e.g., an acute depressive or manic episode). Typically, the medication has already been proven effective in RCTs in the acute phases of illness; the question is whether it is effective for maintenance treatment. If a patient responds (e.g., for the acute mood episode), he/she enters the RCT that tests whether he/she will stay well by remaining on that medication, as opposed to having it stopped (whether receiving placebo or active control). Thereby, for patients who respond to a drug in an initial nonrandomized phase of acute treatment, enriched RCTs test whether they continue to respond.

From the FDA perspective (FDA 2019), enrichment is seen as having three potential uses:

1. "Practical" enrichment, which produces a more homogeneous sample, thus reducing statistical "noise."
2. "Predictive" enrichment, which produces a more treatment responsive sample, thereby increasing effect size.
3. "Prognostic" enrichment, which produces a sample more likely to have the desired outcome (identifying high-risk subjects who are more likely to have the outcome to be measured).

All three strategies should enhance statistical power, allowing for more efficient, ethical, and cost-effective clinical trials.

This critique applies mainly to the second type of *predictive* enrichment, which is the most common use of this design strategy in the psychiatric setting. My view is that, while the other two types of enrichment are likely valid, certain types of predictive enrichment are prone to produce scientifically questionable results and, when used as the basis of FDA indication, could pose public health risks.

Independent Versus Dependent Predictors

For FDA indication purposes, RDTs appear to be most extensively used in psychiatric illnesses, but published RDT studies also are found in oncology, neurology, and immunology, among other fields. For instance, estrogen-receptor-positive tumors are more responsive to drug treatments that affected that receptor, such as tamoxifen. It thus made sense to design studies in which patients were initially preselected as estrogen-receptor-positive, and then randomized to receive tamoxifen or placebo (Fisher et al. 1989). Similarly, a population of patients with high renin status would be expected to be more responsive to an ACE inhibitor antihypertensive agent versus placebo (FDA 2019).

Such predictors are *independent* of the treatment being studied. For instance, an individual may be estrogen-receptor-positive or negative; this fact has nothing to do with whether that person receives tamoxifen or not in a randomized trial. In FDA simulation analyses of oncology designs, RDTs have been seen as most valid and efficient when assessing this kind of independent predictor, viz. molecular targets that are sensitive to chemotherapeutic agents in a subset of tumors (Freidlin and Simon 2005).

Another kind of independently predictive RDT is when the predictor is different than the outcome. A classic example is the important negative Cardiovascular Arrhthymia Suppression Trial (CAST) of drugs proven to acutely suppress paroxysmal ventricular contractions (PVCs) (Ruskin 1989). A subsample of subjects who initially responded to such agents with >70% PVC reduction were randomized to continue drug or switch to placebo, with mortality as the primary outcome – a different outcome than the preselected predictor. Surprisingly to some, the anti-arrhythmic agents increased mortality, a negative outcome.

Such independent predictive RDTs can be either positive or negative, and are informative either way. Unfortunately, even in oncology and cardiology, and certainly in psychiatry, predictive biological markers are often unknown, and hence enrichment in RDTs based on independent predictors is not possible.

When independent biological predictors are not known, it has been proposed that the response to treatment by the test drug can be the predictor for enrichment to (further) assess drug treatment response (Rosner, Stadler, and Ratain 2002). Thereby, a predictor that is known to be *dependent* on the outcome is used: treatment response is used to identify treatment response. The only way this approach could be nontautological would be if the specific type of treatment response was different between predictor and outcome, namely *acute* treatment response (treatment of a *current* episode) as a predictor of *maintenance* treatment response (prevention of future *new* episodes). Posed clinically, this design answers the following question: if a patient initially responds to a medication, will that patient continue to respond to that medication in long-term treatment?

Dependent Predictor and Outcome: Are They the Same?

The use of the dependent predictor of acute treatment response to measure the outcome of maintenance treatment response raises a question of validity: Are predictor and outcome the same? If so, this variety of the RDT design would be statistically invalid.

In psychiatric conditions for which RDTs are used, primarily mood illnesses, the underlying illnesses are remitting and relapsing, not chronic. Mood episodes come and go; they tend not to come and stay unchangingly or worsen unremittingly. Chronic constant depression lasting even one year is rare, occurring in less than 10% of unselected mood illness populations (Goodwin and Jamison 2007). In some of the early RDT proposals in oncology, the context of a progressive chronic disease was taken for granted. RDTs in those studies involved cancers that always worsened, gradually and inexorably. Spontaneous remission was rare.

This difference may be a key feature to understanding why RDTs may be being misused in providing FDA indications in psychiatry.

Most psychiatric studies of maintenance treatment have involved drugs that have been repeatedly proven effective in acute disease states versus placebo, and then they are tested in RDT samples of patients in whom the acute response is confirmed. These studies are invariably positive in the putative maintenance outcome. For instance, an FDA analysis found that all *maintenance* RDTs of antidepressants in MDD over the past 25 years have claimed efficacy (14/14 studies; Borges et al. 2014), while only about half (38/74 studies) of acute classical nonenriched RCTs of antidepressants for *acute* depression in MDD showed efficacy (Turner et al. 2008).

One reason for this outcome may be that the apparent maintenance outcome is merely a reassessment of the acute phase outcome. In other words, the same outcome is being measured twice: once before randomization (when acute nonrandomized responders are selected), and again after randomization (when those taken off the acutely effective drug relapse back into the acute phase). The failure to measure a different outcome, prevention of a new episode in the maintenance phase, is suggested by the rapid relapse of most patients in psychiatric RDTs. The natural history of the acute phase of depressive episodes is that they tend to last 3–6 months in bipolar illness and 6–12 months in unipolar depression (Goodwin and Jamison 2007). The majority of relapses in RDTs of those conditions occur in the first 6 months after the study begins – that is, after treatment of the acute phase to initial response (Goodwin, Whitham, and Ghaemi 2011). Typically, the nonrandomized treatment of the enriched acute phase (before the RDT of the purported maintenance phase begins) occurs for about two months (range up to four months). Thus, most relapses are occurring in RDTs just a few months into an acute mood episode, which is still within the natural history of the acute phase of illness. New episodes occurring 6–12 months later are infrequently observed in RDTs (Goodwin, Whitham, and Ghaemi 2011), and the drug efficacy is driven mostly by early relapses in the first 6 months of follow-up – that is, NOT in the maintenance phase.

In other words, psychiatric RDTs are tautologous in what they measure: they preselect patients for acute response, then they measure acute response again (but they label it "maintenance response").

Hence, it may not be surprising to note that there are few (if any) studies of a drug that is effective in an acute disease state, which is then given for maintenance treatment in a RDT design, in which the result has been negative. We identified only 1 potential case in psychiatric studies (a study of ECT) (Kellner et al. 2006) out of at least 30 such studies in unipolar and bipolar illness as well as schizophrenia (Goodwin, Whitham, and Ghaemi 2011; El-Mallakh and Briscoe 2012; Leucht et al. 2012; Borges et al. 2014). Since a valid scientific design should be falsifiable (Popper 1959), the infrequency of negative studies raise questions about the RDT design's validity.

The Inverse Enriched Design

One can see how the RDT design can mistakenly suggest drug efficacy rather than spontaneous recovery if RDTs in unipolar depressive illness are examined in what might be called a "reverse" enriched design, whereby study populations are enriched with placebo responders. Patients treated acutely who respond to placebo stay on placebo, or are switched to antidepressant, for the maintenance phase. In seven RDTs with such data available, there is *more* maintenance depressive relapse with antidepressant (42%) versus placebo (25%) (Andrews PW 2011). Should we conclude that placebo is more effective than antidepressant in maintenance treatment of unipolar depression? If one reverses the terms, in the standard RDT analysis of antidepressant maintenance efficacy in those preselected to respond to antidepressants, antidepressants are more effective than placebo in the maintenance phase (Geddes et al. 2003). Presumably the reverse enriched RDT design preselects for patients who will do well on placebo, perhaps because they have a more spontaneously recovering illness. However, this may not mean that placebo is inherently more effective than drug. Similarly, the standard enriched RDT design preselects for patients who will do well on a drug that is effective acutely, at least for some time in the continuation phase of treatment. However, this equally may not mean that drug is inherently more effective than placebo. Which enriched RDT analysis is valid: the one enriched for placebo, or the one enriched for antidepressant? It seems apparent that the RDT analysis cannot adjudicate efficacy in the scenario of a spontaneously recovering illness such as unipolar depression.

Rejoinder

A rejoinder that has been made to the foregoing analysis is that acute response will not predict maintenance response since acute "responders" include some patients who would have gotten better anyway (are not responding to the pharmacological properties of the agent): so-called "placebo responders."

A reply to this critique is that so-called "placebo responders" still only represent a proportion of response to drugs which are proven to be more effective than placebo in acute treatment. For instance, if olanzapine produces 60% acute response for acute mania, and placebo produces 40% acute response (these are typical effect sizes), then 40% of the absolute "olanzapine" response involves placebo responders. But 20% of the absolute "olanzapine" response is actually response to that drug pharmacologically; in relative size, this is 1/3 (20%/60%) of the acute olanzapine responders. So, a RDT enriched for olanzapine response will be biased by a factor of 1/3 in favor of olanzapine. This bias can be sufficient to produce a positive response in the RDT withdrawal paradigm. In other words, even allowing for "placebo responders," the RDT design will still be biased in favor of an acutely responsive drug.

Statistical Power

If RDTs produce a more homogeneous sample, fewer subjects would be exposed to the usual ethical risks of RCTs, especially in long-term outcomes that include the use of placebo (Fava et al. 2003). In one of the original simulation models of the RDT design, it was estimated that samples could be utilized that were 20–50% smaller than in standard parallel-design RCTs (Kopec, Abrahamowicz, and Esdaile 1993) with similar recent simulation results (Karrison et al. 2012).

But the assumption of increased power becomes dubious if the validity of the RDT design itself is questionable, as described earlier. The issue of power could then be posed another way: would RDTs increase power so much that they might inflate effect sizes such that a null effect size could no longer be detected? This would threaten the validity of the design in general. The only psychiatric drug in which this inflation effect can be estimated, because of the presence of both enriched and nonenriched studies, is lithium. In nonenriched maintenance studies, lithium efficacy for bipolar disorder ranged from odds ratios (ORs) of 1.9 [95% CIs 1.2–2.8] (newer studies, n = 638) to 3.2 [95% CIs 0.6–15.5] (older trials, n = 130). For three enriched trials (n = 252), a huge pooled OR of 22.0 [95% CIs 7.0–68.7] was found, corresponding to 7–10-fold higher effect estimates than were observed in the nonenriched designs (Deshauer et al. 2005). The question would thus be: Assuming the true effect size was the null, would an enriched design automatically produce an odds ratio of 7–10?

The Case of Lamotrigine

There is one apparent exception to the critique of the validity of RDTs in the psychiatric literature. The anticonvulsant lamotrigine has been shown to be *ineffective* in multiple acute studies of depressive and manic episodes, yet it was effective in RDTs of mood episodes in bipolar disorder (Ghaemi 2009). In our analysis, such maintenance RDT efficacy in an acutely ineffective drug is no different than simply randomizing such patients, without prior enrichment, in a classic RCT. The RDT in that case is more expensive and unnecessarily complicated because it initially excludes a large subsample of acute "nonresponders" who might have "responded" (for prevention of new episodes) later in the maintenance phase.

In sum, if there is positive response in acute use, RDTs appear mostly, if not always, positive, raising questions about their validity. If there is no acute response, then RDTs have no advantage over a traditional nonenriched RCT design.

Phase II Versus Phase III Validity

It is worthwhile distinguishing the assumptions that underlie RDTs in oncology as opposed to in psychiatry. In oncology, the view is that those tumors that do not respond acutely to a chemotherapeutic agent are unlikely to respond in longer-term treatment because those subjects would be a treatment-refractory subgroup (Capra 2004). Similar considerations apply to chronic conditions like cystic fibrosis and degenerative joint disease. In psychiatry, study designs used for mood illnesses would not necessarily pick out subgroups with "advanced disease," or unresponsive to further treatment. In fact, mood-stabilizing agents, like lithium and lamotrigine, are well known to have less benefit in acute treatment of mood episodes, despite showing marked benefit in longer-term prevention of future mood episodes (Ghaemi 2009).

Further, in oncology, RDT designs are mainly advocated for Phase II studies, not Phase III trials (Sharma, Stadler, and Ratain 2011). RDTs are seen as better alternatives for finding a suggestion of treatment benefit than options such open-label studies or historical controls. RDTs are not seen as definitive demonstrations of efficacy, but a kind of advanced pilot testing for definitive classic RCTs. A similar use was made in cardiology with a small 38-subject placebo-controlled RDT of nifedipine for vasospastic angina (Schick et al. 1982).

In psychiatry, in contrast, with the exception of schizophrenia studies, Phase III protocols of maintenance efficacy in the last two decades have consisted mostly of nothing but

RDTs. Most of these studies have involved agents for depression or bipolar disorder (i.e., mood illnesses). FDA indications have ensued for a number of agents (among antipsychotics: olanzapine, aripiprazole, and quetiapine for bipolar disorder; among anticonvulsants: lamotrigine for bipolar disorder; among antidepressants: venlafaxine, paroxetine, atomoxetine, fluoxetine, among others).

Practical Aspects: Feasibility, Cost, and Withdrawal Effects

Early uses of RDTs as approved by the FDA in past decades might have been supported on the practical basis that so few psychotropic agents were available for certain indications, such as maintenance treatment of bipolar disorder, so more efficient clinical trial designs, like RDTs, were justified. But now that multiple drugs are FDA-approved for all phases of mood illnesses, this justification seems less relevant for those indications. Further, as noted, RDTs, if valid, would seem most defensible in Phase II studies, rather than definitive Phase III studies, as they are currently accepted by the FDA for psychiatric indications.

Because of increased power or inflated effect sizes, it is also judged that RDTs are more cost-efficient to conduct. Especially in psychiatry, it is claimed that patients are difficult to study and large samples are both infeasible and expensive, so the enriched design allows for demonstration of efficacy in a feasible and affordable manner (Bowden et al. 1997). Psychiatric patients may be more difficult to study than patients with other medical illnesses, but recent enriched maintenance designs have begun to demonstrate the ability to enroll large samples. For instance, there were 2,503 subjects in 3 studies of the antipsychotic quetiapine for bipolar disorder (Vieta et al. 2008; Suppes et al. 2009; Weisler et al. 2011). If those studies had been nonenriched, even larger samples could have been studied, as 5,852 participants were recruited overall for open acute treatment, but then 56% who were nonresponders were excluded from the maintenance RDT phase. These sample sizes, studied for up to one year, compare favorably with the size of typical RCTs of other types of medications (Table 20.1). The notion that the pharmaceutical industry cannot bear the cost of large studies is somewhat undermined by the fact that some psychiatric medications, like antipsychotic agents, are similar to many statin agents in worldwide profitability (IMS 2011). Further, standard RCTs may save costs by not needing to recruit and then exclude large numbers of patients in the enrichment phase of RDTs.

A final practical limitation to RDTs, at least in the psychiatric setting, is that they commonly produce withdrawal effects and high dropout rates, with more than 90% of patients dropping out at 1–2 years of follow-up (sometimes 100% of patients drop out; see Table 20.1 for comparison of enriched antipsychotic studies with a nonenriched classical RCT of an antihypertensive drug) (Goodwin 2011). Such extremely high dropout rates make maintenance study results difficult to interpret. It is notable that one of the few contemporary psychiatric nonenriched RCT maintenance studies, a two-year comparison of lithium versus valproate in prevention of bipolar disorder (the BALANCE trial) (Geddes et al. 2010), had a low dropout rate (23%), similar to or better than antihypertensive trials.

Clinical Assumptions: Acute Versus Maintenance Response

The main clinical claim for the RDT design is that it tests whether a drug that is effective for acute use should be continued or not, and for how long. It is unclear whether the RDT design answers this question any better than a classic RCT.

Table 20.1 Comparison of RCTs versus RDTs in cardiology and psychiatry: Trial considerations

Studies	Sample size	Enrichment	Mean follow-up (months)	Maximum study duration (years)	Dropouts at 2 years (%)	Number of sites	Concomitant medications allowed*
CHARM Candersartan (2003)	7,599	No	37.7	3.5	43	628	Yes
QTP as adjunct to lithium/VPA US study (2009)	628	Yes	6.2	2	96	127	No
QTP as adjunct to VPA Europe Study (2008)	706	Yes	6.3	2	96	177	No
QTP monotherapy (2011)	1,172	Yes	3.0	1	100	193	No

* For treatment of the primary illness (i.e., hypertension or mania/depression), as opposed to peripherally relevant medications (i.e., hypnotics for sleep). QTP: quetiapine; VPA: valproic acid; **Number of patients are not only in the above-mentioned maintenance trials, but include all major candersartan RCTs and all quetiapine RCTs in acute bipolar depression and major depressive disorder studies.

Table 20.2 Relationship between acute and maintenance response

	Acute response	Acute nonresponse
Maintenance response	A	B
Maintenance nonresponse	C	D

In acute nonresponse scenarios (B and D), classical RCTs have the same validity and greater statistical power than RDTs (no patients are excluded after initial treatment, there are no withdrawal effects, and there are fewer dropouts).

In acute response scenarios, classical RCTs have greater validity than RDTs in scenario C (RDTs rarely, if ever, demonstrate maintenance nonresponse after acute response). RDTs have greater statistical power than RCTs only in scenario A.

In sum: RCTs have more statistical power than RDTs in 2 of 4 scenarios, RDTs have more statistical power than RCTs in one scenario, and RCTs are of equal or greater validity than RDTs in all scenarios.

Clinicians sometimes seem to assume that acute treatment response necessarily implies maintenance response. But counterexamples are common in medicine: indomethacin is an acute treatment for gout but not maintenance, while allopurinol is effective maintenance treatment but not effective (indeed, counterproductive) for acute use; sumatriptan is an acute treatment for migraine but not maintenance, penicillin can treat acute pneumonia but is poor at maintenance prophylaxis; steroids are much more effective for acute episodes of auto-immune illnesses than for prophylaxis. Lithium and lamotrigine are much more effective in prevention of mood episodes of bipolar illness than in treatment of acute episodes (Goodwin and Jamison 2007). In a large NIMH-sponsored study, antidepressants are about twice as effective in treating acute depressive episodes than in preventing them (Rush et al. 2006a).

Hence, an equivalence between acute and maintenance efficacy needs to be proven; it cannot be assumed. There appear to be four logical possibilities, as shown in Table 20.2.

In the case of acute response to a drug, RDTs have greater statistical power in one scenario (A), where the drug is effective in both the acute and the maintenance phases of treatment. In scenario B, where an acutely effective drug is in fact ineffective for mainten-ance treatment, RDTs that are designed based on preselecting acute drug responders are less valid than classic RCTs for the reasons given in this chapter (e.g., withdrawal effects, highly infrequent or absent negative studies, high dropout rates).

In the case of acute nonresponse to a drug (scenarios B and D), classical RCTs have greater statistical power than RDTs (initial treated sample that is nonresponsive is excluded in RDTs but included in RCTs, there are more dropouts in RDTs, and more withdrawal relapses in RDTs).

In sum: RCTs have more statistical power than RDTs in two of four scenarios, RDTs have more statistical power than RCTs in one scenario, and RCTs are of equal or greater validity than RDTs in all scenarios.

RDTs: Going Backward on Generalizability

This analysis of the limitations of RDTs, both in validity and efficiency, relates to an increasing appreciation that "efficacy trials" on highly selected participants are less helpful, because of their lack of generalizability and applicability to usual care, than "effectiveness trials." In addition to aiming to make trials closer to the effectiveness model, one possible approach is integrated efficacy-to-effectiveness (E2E) clinical trials (Selker et al. 2013), whereby initially more restrictive RCT efficacy designs are later broadened, as part of the same study, to assess outcomes in more generalizable samples.

Whatever approach is taken, there is a consensus in the clinical trial community that traditional randomized efficacy trials do not provide enough clinically useful information for usual medical practice. RDTs are a step in the opposite direction, with even less generalizable results (and also diminished validity) than usual efficacy trials. Some investigators have even proposed extending the RDT approach from maintenance studies to acute trials in psychiatry (Fava et al. 2003). This approach, which has received support from the FDA, would appear to head the psychiatric field in the wrong direction, in terms of both validity and generalizability.

Hence, a reconsideration of RDTs should be undertaken in the context of this general trend, apparent in most of medicine other than psychiatry, toward recognizing a need for less, rather than more, preselection and manipulation of samples in randomized drug trials.

Conclusions

This summary of two decades of experience with RDTs suggests that they appear most valid when used with (a) an independent predictor of treatment response (such as a known biological marker), and/or (b) a chronic, progressive disease, without frequent episodic recovery. If the first criterion of an independent marker is absent, RDTs should be used primarily as Phase II pilot studies in preparation for larger classical RCTs for definitive determination of drug efficacy. The current state of antipsychotic, anticonvulsant, and antidepressant maintenance research in psychiatric indications – primarily mood illnesses – does not meet the proposed criteria. Changes in FDA policy would help better establish true drug efficacy in these psychiatric settings, ending its sole reliance on RDTs and requiring a return to some usage of traditional nonenriched RCT designs with larger samples and longer durations of treatment than are currently required.

Such classical RCTs can be conducted in ways that are practically feasible, more efficient, and have as much (if not more) statistical power than RDTs. Most importantly, if this analysis is correct, such RCTs are more scientifically valid than RDTs as currently conducted in psychiatric maintenance studies. Clinical practice for long-term psychiatric treatment, as currently based on potentially invalid RDT designs, would then be based on more valid scientific assessments of long-term efficacy and thus expose the large population of patients who receive these agents to risks and side effects only where these medications are proven effective at a level of scientific validity that is consistent with the rest of medical practice.

Appendix: Understanding Regression

This appendix provides more detail on statistical methods to reduce confounding bias in observational studies, focusing on two main approaches: stratification and regression.

Stratification

Stratification means that one sees how patients do with and without the potential confounder. With the example of a study of whether a toxin causes cancer, it is important to know how many smokers and nonsmokers there are in the sample. If the toxin causes the same cancer rate in smokers as it does in nonsmokers, then you can conclude that smoking does not explain the results. Similarly, in a study of antidepressant treatment of bipolar disorder, for instance, one could assess the results in those with rapid cycling and separately in those without rapid cycling. If the survival curves all had the same results, then one could conclude that it would be unlikely that rapid cycling was a confounder. The advantage of stratification is that it is easy to interpret and does not require complex statistics. The disadvantage is that one can really only look at one confounder at a time.

Stratification is a markedly underused method of addressing confounding bias (Rothman and Greenland 1998). At a simple level, if two strata on a potential confounding factor (e.g., smoking) are the same, then that factor *cannot* confound one's results. Further, if a study does not contain any (or hardly any) persons with a potential confounding factor, then it *cannot* be confounded by that factor (this is called "restriction," as opposed to "stratification").

One of the benefits of stratification, compared to regression, is that one does not need to make certain assumptions about whether the regression model can be applied to the data. The key weakness is that one cannot correct for multiple confounders simultaneously, but at least one can capture major confounders with this simple method. Also, one can use stratification to do sensitivity analyses, looking at whether individual factors change one's results.

Regression

What if, as is usually the case, one thinks there might be multiple confounders? For instance, besides rapid cycling, what if we are concerned about differences in severity of illness, or gender, age, or even things like the therapeutic alliance, or patient compliance, or other factors? Stratification does not handle more than one or a few confounders at a time. For multiple confounders, one has to use a mathematical process called a *regression* model.

To ease the potential strangeness of such statistical language to clinicians, it is important to note that regression models basically represent the same thing (quantified) that clinicians do intuitively. When clinicians see patients, they conceive of patients in terms of the whole complexity of the presentation. Thus, one patient might be an elderly, obese male with medical illness and many side effects who has been unwell for decades. Another patient might be a young, thin female with no previous treatment and only a short period of illness. Even in these simple clinical descriptions, multiple factors (age, gender, duration of illness, past treatment response, weight) are intuitively taken into account by experienced clinicians as they make judgments about diagnosis and treatment. Regression models simply identify and quantify the effects of these clinical factors on outcome.

The key to regression is that it allows one to measure the experimental effect adjusted for some of the confounders. It also allows one to get the magnitude of effect of the various predictors on their own. The main disadvantage of regression models is that they do not control or adjust for confounders for which one may not have accurate or adequate data, nor do they adjust for potential confounders that are unknown at the time of the study. These latter problems are only addressed by randomization. But, in the setting of observational studies, regression modeling can reduce, though never completely remove, confounding bias.

Conflicting Studies

A major reason why conflicting studies are present in the treatment literature of bipolar disorder is that many of those studies are observational studies, and the vast majority make no effort to identify or correct for confounding bias. As Hill wrote, "One difficulty, in view of the variability of patients and their illnesses, is in classifying the patients into, at least, broad groups so that we may be sure that like is put with like, both before and after treatment" (Hill 1971, p. 9). When confounding bias is not assessed in observational studies, often like is not being compared with like, and all kinds of varying results will be reported.

Assessing Confounding Factors

How should one compare two groups to tell whether differences between them might reflect confounding bias? Two basic options exist: to use p-values, or simply to compare the magnitude of difference between the groups. Computer simulation models have compared these alternatives and, all in all, the magnitude of difference approach seems most sensitive to detecting confounding effects. p-Values are too coarse of a measure: they only capture major differences between groups (if they are used, the computer simulations suggest that they should be set at a high level; for example, $p < 0.20$ would indicate a difference that could lead to potential confounding effects). However, two subgroups in a sample may have a moderate or even small difference on some factor, but if that factor has a major effect on the outcome, a confounding effect can happen. In the computer simulations, it was found that a low potential absolute difference between groups (such as 10%) predicted confounding effects rather well.

The Meaning of "Adjusted" Data

In sum, the basic concept behind regression modeling is that we will control for all potential confounding variables. In other words, we will look at the results for the variable which interests us (one might call it the *experimental* variable), *while keeping all other variables fixed*. So, if we want to know whether antidepressants cause mania, the outcome is mania and the experimental variable is antidepressant use. If we want to remove the effect of other confounding variables – such as age, gender, age of onset, years ill, severity of depression, etc. – we will put those variables into a regression model. The mathematical equation of the regression model can be seen, in a way, as keeping all those other values fixed, so as to give a more accurate result for the experimental variable (antidepressant use). The outcome of looking at antidepressant use and mania without assessing other confounding variables is called the *unadjusted* or *crude* result. The outcome of assessing antidepressant use and mania while also controlling for other confounding variables is called the *adjusted* result. Another way of putting this process is that we are adjusting the results which appear to be the case at face value (the *crude* results) to make them closer to what they *really* are (or what they really would be seen to be in a randomized study, where the effect of all confounding variables is removed). If the crude (or unadjusted) and the adjusted results are not much different, then the variables included in the model did not have much confounding effect. In that case, the crude results can be seen as valid – unless, of course, one has failed to identify some variables which might have exerted confounding effects and that are not adjusted in the regression model.

A Conceptual Defense of Regression

Some people do not like the concept of adjustment, perhaps because it smacks of fiddling with the data: after all, the "real" results, what are actually observed, are being mathematically manipulated. Such critics fail to realize that *what one observes in the real world is often not what is really there.* This is another philosophical concept, which is simple to show to be true, at the basis of statistics. The sun appears to be about the size of my hand, but it is much larger. I have never seen an atom, but this apparently solid table is made of them. What appears to be the case is not all there is to reality. So it is with clinical observations in medicine. We think coffee causes cancer if we simply associate the two, but the coffee drinkers are also smokers and the cause is the latter. If we do not assess smoking and take it into account, the "real" observation of coffee and cancer will fool us.

Hence, adjustment in regression models is perfectly legitimate, but the phrase can be altered, if one prefers, to variants such as "controlling" for confounding factors or "correcting" for confounding factors. Any of these terms are interchangeable: "adjusted" results, or results "controlled" or "corrected" for other variables.

Regression Equations

The mathematical concept behind regression modeling is complex, but the basics are worth understanding since results are often reported with the basic equation's terms.

If I want to know the probability of an association between an experimental predictor (as defined earlier) and an outcome, I can express it simply this way:

P (Outcome) = B (Predictor)

Where P (Outcome) = the probability of the outcome

And B (Predictor) = the effect of the predictor.

B is the variable for the effect size of the predictor, or how much the predictor impacts on the outcome.

As described in Chapter 9, effect sizes come in two varieties: absolute and relative. Absolute effect sizes are amounts, such as the difference between drug and placebo on a mood rating scale. If drug leads to 5 points more improvement on the rating scale than placebo, then the *absolute effect size* between the two treatments is 5. Effect size can also be relative. If 80% of those on drug improved markedly versus 20% of those on placebo, then the relative effect size is 80/20 = 4. This is often called the *risk ratio*, a type of relative risk. Another kind of relative risk is the *odds ratio*, which is another way of expressing the risk ratio. While the straight risk ratio is a probability, the odds ratio is a measure of a fair bet that something will happen. Thus, with a die, the chances are 1/6 that any one number will happen. But the odds are 5 to 1. Thus, in our example, a risk ratio of 4 means one group is 4 times more likely to have the result. However, if one wishes to place a bet on the outcome in Las Vegas, one can say the same thing by saying that the odds are 16 to 1 that this result would occur. Hence, odds ratios and risk ratios are different, and as probabilities increase for risk ratios, odds ratios increase exponentially.

The relevance of this discussion is that the relative effect sizes that are obtained in regression models are odds ratios, not risk ratios, and thus we need to remember that huge odds do not represent absolute probabilities of that size. The equation for regression models involves logarithms, and the conversion of logarithms to effect sizes produces odds ratios, not risk ratios.

Multivariate Regression

Back to our equation. We have a predictor and an outcome; this is an association which is direct and uncorrected for any potential confounding variables. In the phrasing of studies, this is a *univariate* analysis; only one predictor is assessed. We might be interested in two predictors, or we might want to adjust our results for one other variable besides our experimental variable. Our equation would then become:

$$P \text{ (Outcome)} = \beta \text{ (Predictor}_1) + \beta \text{ (Predictor}_2)$$

where Predictor$_1$ is the experimental variable, and Predictor$_2$ is the second variable, which might be a confounding factor, or which might itself be a second predictor of the outcome. This equation is a *bivariate* analysis.

Sometimes researchers report bivariate analyses, comparing the experimental with the outcome, correcting for a single variable, *one after the other, separately*. This would be something like:

$$P \text{ (Outcome)} = \beta \text{ (Predictor}_1) + \beta \text{ (Predictor}_2)$$
$$P \text{ (Outcome)} = \beta \text{ (Predictor}_1) + \beta \text{ (Predictor}_3)$$
$$P \text{ (Outcome)} = \beta \text{ (Predictor}_1) + \beta \text{ (Predictor}_4)$$
$$P \text{ (Outcome)} = \beta \text{ (Predictor}_1) + \beta \text{ (Predictor}_5)$$

The problem with these bivariate analyses is that they will correct the experimental predictor for each one separately, but they do not correct it for *all variables together*. Let us suppose that the experimental predictor is coffee drinking and the outcome is cancer; and let us suppose that the main confounding factor is smoking but that this effect is primarily seen in older smokers rather than younger smokers. Thus, the confounding effect involves two variables: smoking and age. If Predictor$_2$ is smoking, and Predictor$_3$ is age, then this combined effect will be underestimated in serial bivariate equations. This effect can only be seen in multivariate analysis, where all the factors are included in one model:

$$P \text{ (Outcome)} = \beta \text{ (Predictor}_1) + \beta \text{ (Predictor}_2) + \beta \text{ (Predictor}_3) + \beta \text{ (Predictor}_4) + \beta \text{ (Predictor}_5)$$

The other benefit of multivariate analysis is that it not only corrects the effect size of the experimental variable β (Predictor$_1$) for the other predictor variables, but it also *corrects all the predictor variables for each other*. Thus, if the estimate of the effect size of the impact of smoking on cancer is confounded by age (higher in older persons and lower in younger persons), then the multivariate analysis will correct for age in the effect size that is estimated for the smoking variable.

Visualizing Regression

We can now perhaps best proceed with understanding regression modeling by visualizing what it entails. Suppose the probability of the outcome – P (Outcome) – is on the y axis, and on the x axis we have the adjusted effect size (β value) of the experimental predictor.

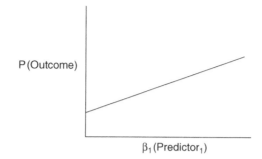

P(Outcome)

β_1(Predictor$_1$)

Figure A.1 Outcome versus Predictor

The graph of this process would look something like what follows:

The slope of this line is the effect size, or β value, with the probability of the outcome varying

Take the example of someone who is age 35 and has been ill with depression for 20 years, in whom we want to assess the efficacy of antidepressants (Predictor$_1$ is antidepressant use and the Outcome is being classified as a treatment responder); the equation would be:

P (Outcome) = β_1 (antidepressant use) + β_2 (age) + β_3 (years ill)

Which would be

P (Outcome) = β_1 (antidepressant use) + β_2 (35) + β_3 (20).

Another patient might have received antidepressant but with an age of 55 and 30 years ill, producing the equation:

P (Outcome) = β_1 (antidepressant use) + β_2 (55) + β_3 (30).

In these cases, the calculation of the effect of antidepressant use, β_1, would be adjusted for, or corrected for, the changes in age and years ill between patients. In other words, β_1 would not change in the above two equations. It is as if the values for the effect of age (β_2) and years ill (β_3) were calculated at an average amount for all patients, or kept constant in all patients, thus removing any differences they might cause in the overall equation.

The differing patients might be visualized as in Figure A.1:

What is visually clear is that the slopes are always the same, that is, the effect size for the experimental predictor – β (Predictor$_1$) – never changes. The change in the absolute result of the equation is only reflected in changes in the y-intercept, which is captured mathematically as β_0, a term which has no relevant clinical meaning but which reflects the start of the curve that is being modeled with regression.

The equation of a multivariate regression model then ends up as follows:

P (Outcome) = β_0 + β_1 (Predictor$_1$) + β_2 (Predictor$_2$) + β_3 (Predictor$_3$) + β_4 (Predictor$_4$) + β_5 (Predictor$_5$) . . ..

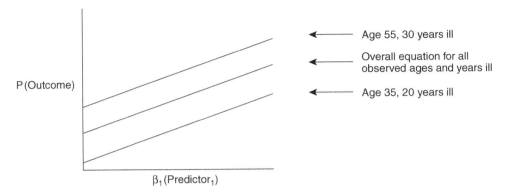

Figure A.2 Outcome versus Predictor₁ adjusted for other predictors (e.g., age, years ill)

Not Too Many Variables

The number of predictors can obviously not be infinite. Researchers need to define how many predictors or confounders need to be included in a regression model. How this process of choice occurs can be somewhat subjective, or it might be put into the hands of a computer model. In either case, some kind of decision must be made, often due to sample size limitations. Mathematically, the more variables that are included in a regression model, the lower the statistical power of the analysis. This is referred to as *collinearity*, since frequently variables will correlate with each other (such as age and number of years ill), and thus multiple variables may in fact be assessing the same clinical predictor. Besides this factor, as noted earlier, multiple statistical comparisons always increase the risks of chance outcomes. (As noted later, this factor is perhaps the major limitation in regression modeling). In other words, even if an experimental variable strongly impacts an outcome in a study of 100 patients, this strong result might be statistically significant in a univariate analysis, a bivariate analysis, or even a multivariate analysis with 5 variables. But if 15 variables are included, eventually that p-value will rise above 0.05, and suddenly – poof, there is no result! We want to avoid saying there is no effect when there might indeed be one, and thus one should not include too many variables in a regression model. But how many is too many? Deciding which variables to include and which to exclude is a complex process.

Effect Modification Again

Readers should be reminded that interactions between predictors and other variables do not always reflect confounding effects; sometimes they reflect effect modification. As discussed in Chapter 4, this is where it is useful, even necessary, to be a clinician: To appreciate confounding bias versus effect modification, one needs to understand the condition and variables being studied. In confounding bias, the confounding variable *is* itself the causal source of the outcome; in effect modification, the effect modifier *is not* the causal source of the outcome (the experimental variable causes the outcome, but only through interaction with the effect modifier). The numbers alone cannot tell this story; the researcher needs to think about the illness.

Recall classic examples from medical epidemiology, repeated here from Chapter 4 so that this distinction is clear. Here is an example of effect modification: Cigarette smoking frequently causes blood clots in women on birth control pills. Being female itself is not a cause of blood clots, nor do oral contraceptives themselves have a large risk, but those two variables (gender and oral contraceptive status) together increase the risk of cigarette smoking greatly. Contrast this example with confounding bias: Coffee causes cancer; numerous epidemiological studies show this. Of course, it does not, because coffee drinking is higher among those who smoke cigarettes, and cigarette smoking (the confounding variable) is the cause of the cancer.

Regression in RCTs

Up to now, to keep it simple, I have emphasized the use of regression modeling only for observational studies. In contrast, I have said that in clinical trials, they are not needed: since confounding bias is removed by the research design (randomization), there is no need to try to remove it by data analysis (regression modeling).

Some take this distinction too literally, thereby creating a fetish out of RCTs (randomized clinical trials). In fact, regression modeling should still be used even after RCTs are conducted as a mechanism of sensitivity analysis. In other words, did those RCTs in fact succeed in removing confounding bias? If they did, then regression models should not change any of the findings about the relationship between experimental variables and outcomes (unlike observational studies). If, however, regression models change some results, then either confounding bias or effect modification might be at work, and the RCT would need to be more carefully analyzed.

This is relevant because even though RCTs are *meant* to remove confounding bias by means of randomization, one cannot assume that they *succeed* in doing so. One cannot *assume* the success of randomization; one must *prove* it.

References

Abramson, J. 2004. *Overdosed America: The Broken Promise of American Medicine* (Harper Collins: New York).

Abramson, J. H., and Z. H. Abramson. 2001. *Making Sense of Data: A Self-Instruction Manual on the Interpretation of Epidemiological Data* (Oxford University Press: New York).

Altshuler, L., T. Suppes, D. Black, et al. 2003. "Impact of antidepressant discontinuation after acute bipolar depression remission on rates of depressive relapse at 1-year follow-up," *Am J Psychiatry*, 160: 1252–62.

Andrews, G., K. Anstey, H. Brodaty, C. Issakidis, and G. Luscombe. 1999. "Recall of depressive episode 25 years previously," *Psychol Med*, 29: 787–91.

Andrews P. W., S. G. Kornstein, L. J. Halberstadt, C. O. Gardner, and M. C. Neale. 2011. "Blue again: Perturbational effects of antidepressants suggest monoaminergic homeostasis in major depression," *Front Psychol*, 2: 1–24.

Angell, M. 2005. *The Truth about the Drug Companies* (Random House: New York).

Bachmann, S. 2018. "Epidemiology of suicide and the psychiatric perspective," *Int J Environ Res Public Health*, 15: 1425.

Barbui, C., A. Cipriani, L. Malvini, and M. Tansella. 2006. "Validity of the impact factor of journals as a measure of randomized controlled trial quality," *J Clin Psychiatry*, 67: 37–40.

Barnard, G. A. , and T. Bayes. 1958. "Studies in the history of probability and statistics: IX. Thomas Bayes's essay Towards Solving a Problem in the Doctrine of Chances," *Biometrika*, 45: 293–315. https://doi.org/10.2307/2333180.

Basoglu, M., I. Marks, M. Livanou, and R. Swinson. 1997. "Double-blindness procedures, rater blindness, and ratings of outcome: Observations from a controlled trial," *Arch Gen Psychiatry*, 54: 744–8.

Baxt, W. G., J. F. Waeckerle, J. A. Berlin, and M. L. Callaham. 1998. "Who reviews the reviewers? Feasibility of using a fictitious manuscript to evaluate peer reviewer performance," *Ann Emerg Med*, 32: 310–7.

Beck, A. T. 2019. "A 60-year evolution of cognitive theory and therapy," *Perspect Psychol Sci*, 14: 16–20.

Benson, K., and A. J. Hartz. 2000. "A comparison of observational studies and randomized, controlled trials," *N Engl J Med*, 342: 1878–86.

Berry, D. A. 1993. "A case for Bayesianism in clinical trials," *Stat Med*, 12: 1377–93.

Blackwelder, W. C. 1982. "'Proving the null hypothesis' in clinical trials," *Control Clin Trials*, 3: 345–53.

Blair-West, G. W., C. H. Cantor, G. W. Mellsop, and M. L. Eyeson-Annan. 1999. "Lifetime suicide risk in major depression: Sex and age determinants," *J Affect Disord*, 55: 171–8.

Blank, A. 2006. "A piece of my mind: Swan's way," *JAMA*, 296: 1041–2.

Bolwig, T. G. 2006. "Psychiatry and the humanities," *Acta Psychiatr Scand*, 114: 381–3.

Borges, S., Y. F. Chen, T. P. Laughren, et al. 2014. "Review of maintenance trials for major depressive disorder: A 25-year perspective from the US Food and Drug Administration," *J Clin Psychiatry*, 75: 205–14.

Bowden, C. L., J. R. Calabrese, G. S. Sachs, et al. 2003. "A placebo-controlled 18-month trial of lamotrigine and lithium maintenance treatment in recently manic or hypomanic patients with bipolar I disorder," *Arch Gen Psychiatry*, 60: 392–400.

Bowden, C. L., A. C. Swann, J. R. Calabrese, et al. 1997. "Maintenance clinical trials in bipolar disorder: Design implications of the divalproex-lithium-placebo study," *Psychopharmacol Bull*, 33: 693–9.

Brazill, K. P., S. Warnick, Jr., and C. White. 2018. "Revisiting the canons of psychiatry: Teaching the fundamentals of CATIE, STAR*D, and STEP-BD to family medicine residents," *Int J Psychiatry Med*, 53: 455–63.

Brown, H. 2007. "How impact factors changed medical publishing – and science," *BMJ*, 334: 561–4.

Calabrese, J. R., C. L. Bowden, G. S. Sachs, et al. 1999. "A double-blind placebo-controlled study of lamotrigine monotherapy in outpatients with bipolar I depression: Lamictal 602 Study Group," *J Clin Psychiatry*, 60: 79–88.

Calabrese, J. R., C. L. Bowden, G. Sachs, et al. 2003. "A placebo-controlled 18-month trial of lamotrigine and lithium maintenance treatment in recently depressed patients with bipolar I disorder," *J Clin Psychiatry*, 64: 1013–24.

Calabrese, J. R., R. F. Huffman, R. L. White, et al. 2008. "Lamotrigine in the acute treatment of bipolar depression: Results of five double-blind, placebo-controlled clinical trials," *Bipolar Disord*, 10: 323–33.

Calabrese, J. R., P. E. Keck, Jr., W. Macfadden, et al. 2005. "A randomized, double-blind, placebo-controlled trial of quetiapine in the treatment of bipolar I or II depression," *Am J Psychiatry*, 162: 1351–60.

Calabrese, J. R., T. Suppes, C. L. Bowden, et al. 2000. "A double-blind, placebo-controlled, prophylaxis study of lamotrigine in rapid-cycling bipolar disorder: Lamictal 614 Study Group," *J Clin Psychiatry*, 61: 841–50.

Capra, W. B. 2004. "Comparing the power of the discontinuation design to that of the classic randomized design on time-to-event endpoints," *Control Clin Trials*, 25: 168–77.

Carroll, B. J. 2004. "Adolescents with depression," *JAMA*, 292: 2577–9.

2006. "Ten rules of academic life: Reflections on the career of an affective disorders researcher," *J Affect Disord*, 92: 7–12.

Cipriani, A., T. A. Furukawa, G. Salanti, et al. 2009. "Comparative efficacy and acceptability of 12 new-generation antidepressants: A multiple-treatments meta-analysis," *Lancet*, 373: 746–58.

Cipriani, A., T. A. Furukawa, G. Salanti, et al. 2018. "Comparative efficacy and acceptability of 21 antidepressant drugs for the acute treatment of adults with major depressive disorder: A systematic review and network meta-analysis," *Lancet*, 391: 1357–66.

Cohen, J. 1994. "The earth is round (p < 0.05)," *Am Psychol*, 49: 997–1003.

Conner, A., D. Azrael, and M. Miller. 2019. "Suicide case-fatality rates in the United States, 2007 to 2014: A nationwide population-based study," *Ann Intern Med*, 171: 885–95.

Das, A. K., M. Olfson, M. J. Gameroff, et al. 2005. "Screening for bipolar disorder in a primary care practice," *JAMA*, 293: 956–63.

Dawson, B., and R. G. Trapp. 2001. *Basic and Clinical Biostatistics* (McGraw-Hill: New York).

Dennett, D. D. 2000. "Postmodernism and truth," in J. Hintikka, S. Neville, E. Sosa, and A. Olsen (eds.), *Proceedings of the 20th World Congress of Philosophy, Volume 8* (Philosophy Documentation Center: Charlottesville, VA), pp. 93–100.

Deshauer, D., D. Fergusson, A. Duffy, J. Albuquerque, and P. Grof. 2005. "Re-evaluation of randomized control trials of lithium monotherapy: A cohort effect," *Bipolar Disord*, 7: 382–7.

DeVito, N. J., and B. Goldacre. 2021. "Evaluation of compliance with legal requirements under the FDA Amendments Act of 2007 for timely registration of clinical trials, data verification, delayed reporting, and trial document submission," *JAMA Intern Med*, 181: 1128–30.

Doll, R. 2002. "Proof of causality: Deduction from epidemiological observation," *Perspect Biol Med*, 45: 499–515.

El-Mallakh, R. and B. Briscoe. 2012 "Studies of long-term use of antidepressants: How should the data from them be interpreted?" *CNS Drugs*, 26: 97–109. https://doi.org/10.2165/11599450-000000000-00000.

Emanuel, E. J., and F. G. Miller. 2001. "The ethics of placebo-controlled trials: A middle ground," *N Engl J Med*, 345: 915–9.

Eysenck, H. J. 1994. "Meta-analysis and its problems," *BMJ*, 309: 789–92.

Fava, M., A. E. Evins, D. J. Dorer, and D. A. Schoenfeld. 2003. "The problem of the placebo response in clinical trials for psychiatric disorders: Culprits, possible remedies, and a novel study design approach," *Psychother Psychosom*, 72: 115–27.

FDA (Food and Drug Administration). 2019. "Guidance for Industry: Enrichment Strategies for Clinical Trials to Support Approval of Human Drugs and Biological Products."Docket number FDA-2012-D-114 5. Issued by Center for Drug Evaluation and Research, Center for Biologics Evaluation and Research. Accessible at www.fda.gov/re gulatory-information/search-fda-guidance-documents/enrichment-strategies-clinical-trials-support-approval-human-drugs-and-biological-products.

Feinstein, A. R. 1977. *Clinical Biostatistics* (Mosby: St. Louis).

Feinstein, A. R. 1995. "Meta-analysis: Statistical alchemy for the 21st century," *J Clin Epidemiol*, 48: 71–9.

Feinstein, A. R. and R. I. Horwitz. 1997. "Problems in the 'evidence' of 'evidence-based medicine,'" *Am. J. Med.*, 103: 529–35. https://doi.org/10.1016/s0002-9343(97) 00244-1.

Fink, M., and M. A. Taylor. 2007. "Electroconvulsive therapy: Evidence and challenges," *JAMA*, 298: 330–2.

2008. "The medical evidence-based model for psychiatric syndromes: Return to a classical paradigm," *Acta Psychiatr Scand*, 117: 81–4.

Fisher, B., J. Costantino, C. Redmond, et al. 1989. "A randomized clinical trial evaluating tamoxifen in the treatment of patients with node-negative breast cancer who have estrogen-receptor-positive tumors," *N Engl J Med*, 320: 479–84.

Fisher, RA. 1947. *The Design of Experiments* (Oliver and Boyd: London).

1971 [1935]. *The Design of Experiments*, 9th edition (Macmillan: New York).

Fletcher, W. 1907. "Rice and beri-beri: Preliminary report on an experiment conducted at the Kuala Lampur Lunatic Asylum," *Lancet*, i: 1776–79.

Fluckiger, C., A. C. Del Re, B. E. Wampold, and A. O. Horvath. 2018. "The alliance in adult psychotherapy: A meta-analytic synthesis," *Psychotherapy (Chic)*, 55: 316–40.

Fluckiger, C., A. C. Del Re, B. E. Wampold, D. Symonds, and A. O. Horvath. 2012. "How central is the alliance in psychotherapy? A multilevel longitudinal meta-analysis," *J Couns Psychol*, 59: 10–17.

Foucault, M. 1994. *The Birth of the Clinic* (Vintage: New York).

Freidlin, B., and R. Simon. 2005. "Evaluation of randomized discontinuation design," *J Clin Oncol*, 23: 5094–8.

Friedman, L. M., C. D. Furberg, and D. L. DeMets. 1998a. *Fundamentals of Clinical Trials* (Springer-Verlag: New York).

Friedman, L. M., C. D. Furberg, and D. L. DeMets. 1998b. *Fundamentals of Clinical Trials*, 3rd edition (Springer: New York).

Geddes, J. R., S. M. Carney, C. Davies, et al. 2003. "Relapse prevention with antidepressant drug treatment in depressive disorders: A systematic review," *Lancet*, 361: 653–61.

Geddes, J. R., G. M. Goodwin, J. Rendell, et al. 2010. "Lithium plus valproate combination therapy versus monotherapy for relapse prevention in bipolar I disorder (BALANCE): A randomised open-label trial," *Lancet*, 375: 385–95.

Gehlbach, S. 2006. *Interpreting the Medical Literature* (McGraw-Hill: New York).

Ghaemi, S. N. 2003. *The Concepts of Psychiatry: A Pluralistic Approach to the Mind and Mental Illness* (Johns Hopkins University Press: Baltimore, MD).

2008. "Toward a Hippocratic psychopharmacology," *Can J Psychiatry*, 53: 189–96.

2009. "The failure to know what isn't known: Negative publication bias with lamotrigine and a glimpse inside peer review," *Evid Based Ment Health*, 12: 65–8.

Ghaemi, S. N., W. S. Gilmer, J. F. Goldberg, et al. 2007. "Divalproex in the treatment of acute bipolar depression: A preliminary double-blind, randomized, placebo-controlled pilot study," *J Clin Psychiatry*, 68: 1840–4.

Ghaemi, S. N., A. A. Shirzadi, and M. M. Filkowski. 2008a. "Publication bias and the pharmaceutical industry: The case of lamotrigine in bipolar disorder," *Medscape J Med*, 9: 211.

Ghaemi, S. N., F. Soldani, and D. J. Hsu. 2003. "Evidence-based pharmacotherapy of bipolar disorder." *Int. J. Neuropsychopharmacol*, 6: 303–8. https://doi.org/10.1017 /S1461145703003626.

Ghaemi, S. N., A. P. Wingo, M. A. Filkowski, and R. J. Baldessarini. 2008b. "Long-term antidepressant treatment in bipolar disorder: Meta-analyses of benefits and risks," *Acta Psychiatr Scand*, 118: 374–56.

Goff, D. C., P. Falkai, W. W. Fleischhacker, et al. 2017. "The long-term effects of antipsychotic medication on clinical course in schizophrenia," *Am J Psychiatry*, 174: 840–49.

Goldberg, J. F., and J. E. Whiteside. 2002. "The association between substance abuse and antidepressant-induced mania in bipolar disorder: A preliminary study," *J Clin Psychiatry*, 63: 791–5.

Goodman, S. N. 1999. "Toward evidence-based medical statistics. 2: The Bayes factor," *Ann Intern Med*, 130: 1005–13.

Goodwin, F. K., and K. R. Jamison. 2007. *Manic Depressive Illness*, 2nd edition (Oxford University Press: New York).

Goodwin, F. K., E. A. Whitham, and S. N. Ghaemi. 2011. "Maintenance treatment study designs in bipolar disorder: Do they demonstrate that atypical neuroleptics (antipsychotics) are mood stabilizers?," *CNS Drugs*, 25: 819–27.

Hammad, T. A., T. Laughren, and J. Racoosin. 2006. "Suicidality in pediatric patients treated with antidepressant drugs," *Arch Gen Psychiatry*, 63: 332–9.

Healy, D. 2001. *The Creation of Psychopharmacology* (Harvard University Press: Cambridge, MA).

Hill, A. B. 1962. *Statistical Methods in Clinical and Preventive Medicine* (Oxford University Press: New York).

1965. "The environment and disease: Association or causation?," *Proc R Soc Med*, 58: 295–300.

1971. *Principles of Medical Statistics* (Oxford University Pres: New York).

Hill, A. B. 1962b. *Statistical Methods in Clinical and Preventive Medicine* (Oxford University Press: New York).

Horton, R. 2002. "The hidden research paper," *JAMA*, 287: 2775–8.

Hrobjartsson, A., and P. C. Gotzsche. 2001. "Is the placebo powerless? An analysis of clinical trials comparing placebo with no treatment," *N Engl J Med*, 344: 1594–602.

Hummer, M., R. Holzmeister, G. Kemmler, et al. 2003. "Attitudes of patients with schizophrenia toward placebo-controlled clinical trials," *J Clin Psychiatry*, 64: 277–81.

Hunt, M. 1997. *How Science Takes Stock: The Story of Meta-Analysis* (Russell Sage Foundation: London).

IMS. 2011. "The use of medicines in the United States: Review of 2010." IMS Institute for Healthcare Informatics: Parsippany, NJ.

Ioannidis, J. P. 2005. "Contradicted and initially stronger effects in highly cited clinical research," *JAMA*, 294: 218–28.

Isacsson, G., and C. L. Rich. 2014. "Antidepressant drugs and the risk of suicide in children and adolescents," *Paediatr Drugs*, 16: 115–22.

Jaeschke, R., G. Guyatt, and D. L. Sackett. 1994. "Users' guides to the medical literature. III. How to use an article about a diagnostic test. A. Are the results of the study valid? Evidence-Based Medicine Working Group," *JAMA*, 271: 389–91.

James, W. 1956 (1897). "Is life worth living?' in, *The Will to Believe and Other Essays in Popular Philosophy* (Dover: New York).

Jaspers, K. 1997 [1959]. *General Psychopathology: Volumes 1 and 2* (Johns Hopkins University Press: Baltimore, MD).

Jefferson, T., P. Alderson, E. Wager, and F. Davidoff. 2002. "Effects of editorial peer review: A systematic review," *JAMA*, 287: 2784–6.

Joffe, R. T., G. M. MacQueen, M. Marriott, and L. T. Young. 2005. "One-year outcome with antidepressant-treatment of bipolar depression," *Acta Psychiatr Scand*, 112: 105–9.

Jureidini, J. N., C. J. Doecke, P. R. Mansfield, et al. 2004. "Efficacy and safety of antidepressants for children and adolescents," *BMJ*, 328: 879–83.

Karrison, T. G., M. J. Ratain, W. M. Stadler, and G. L. Rosner. 2012. "Estimation of progression-free survival for all treated patients in the randomized discontinuation trial design," *Am Stat*, 66: 155–62.

Katz, I. R., M. P. Rogers, R. Lew, et al. 2022. "Lithium treatment in the prevention of repeat suicide-related outcomes in veterans with major depression or bipolar disorder: A randomized clinical trial," *JAMA Psychiatry*, 79: 24–32.

Kellner, C. H., R. G. Knapp, G. Petrides, et al. 2006. "Continuation electroconvulsive therapy vs pharmacotherapy for relapse prevention in major depression: A multisite study from the Consortium for Research in Electroconvulsive Therapy (CORE)," *Arch Gen Psychiatry*, 63: 1337–44.

Kirsch, I., B. J. Deacon, T. B. Huedo-Medina, et al. 2008. "Initial severity and antidepressant benefits: A meta-analysis of data submitted to the Food and Drug Administration," *PLoS Med*, 5: e45.

Kopec, J. A., M. Abrahamowicz, and J. M. Esdaile. 1993. "Randomized discontinuation trials: Utility and efficiency," *J Clin Epidemiol*, 46: 959–71.

Kraemer, H. C. and D. J. Kupfer. (2006) "Size of treatment effects and their importance to clinical research and practice," *Biol Psychiatry* 59: 990–6.

Krupnick, J. L., S. M. Sotsky, S. Simmens, et al. 1996. "The role of the therapeutic alliance in psychotherapy and pharmacotherapy outcome: Findings in the National Institute of Mental Health Treatment of Depression Collaborative Research Program," *J Consult Clin Psychol*, 64: 532–9.

Kushner, S. F., A. Khan, R. Lane, and W. H. Olson. 2006. "Topiramate monotherapy in the management of acute mania: Results of four double-blind placebo-controlled trials," *Bipolar Disord*, 8: 15–27.

Lang, J. M., K. J. Rothman, and C. I. Cann. 1998. "That confounded P-value," *Epidemiology*, 9: 7–8.

Leon, A. C. 2004. "Multiplicity-adjusted sample size requirements: A strategy to maintain statistical power with Bonferroni adjustments," *J Clin Psychiatry*, 65: 1511–4.

Leucht, S., M. Tardy, K. Komossa, et al. 2012. "Maintenance treatment with antipsychotic drugs for schizophrenia," *Cochrane Database Syst Rev*, 5: CD008016.

Levine, R., and M. Fink. 2006. "The case against evidence-based principles in psychiatry," *Med Hypotheses*, 67: 401–10.

Lexchin, J., L. A. Bero, B. Djulbegovic, and O. Clark. 2003. "Pharmaceutical industry sponsorship and research outcome and quality: Systematic review," *BMJ*, 326: 1167–70.

Mack, JE. 1995. *Abduction: Human Encounters with Aliens* (Ballantine: New York).

Makkreel, R. 1992. *Dilthey: Philosopher of the Human Studies* (Princeton University Press: Princeton, NJ).

Mann, J. J., G. Emslie, R. J. Baldessarini, et al. 2006. "ACNP Task Force report on SSRIs and suicidal behavior in youth," *Neuropsychopharmacol : Off Publ Am Coll Neuropsychopharmacol*, 31: 473–92. https://doi.org/10.1038/sj.npp.1300958.

Manwani, S. G., T. B. Pardo, M. J. Albanese, et al. 2006. "Substance use disorder and other predictors of antidepressant-induced mania: A retrospective chart review," *J Clin Psychiatry*, 67: 1341–5.

March, J., S. Silva, S. Petrycki, et al. 2004. "Fluoxetine, cognitive-behavioral therapy, and their combination for adolescents with depression: Treatment for Adolescents With Depression Study (TADS) randomized controlled trial," *JAMA*, 292: 807–20.

Marcus, R. N., R. D. McQuade, W. H. Carson, et al. 2008. "The efficacy and safety of aripiprazole as adjunctive therapy in major depressive disorder: A second multicenter, randomized, double-blind, placebo-controlled study," *J Clin Psychopharmacol*, 28: 156–65.

Martin, D. J., J. P. Garske, and M. K. Davis. 2000. "Relation of the therapeutic alliance with outcome and other variables: A meta-analytic review," *J Consult Clin Psychol*, 68: 438–50.

McHugh, P. R. 1996. "Hippocrates a la mode," *Nat Med*, 2: 507–9.

Menand, L. 2001. *The Metaphysical Club* (Farrar, Strauss, and Giroux: New York).

Miettinen, O. S. and E. F. Cook. 1981. "Confounding: Essence and detection," *Am J Epidemiol*, 114: 593–603.

Mills, C. W. 1963. *Power, Politics, and People* (Oxford University Press: New York).

Moncrieff, J., S. Wessely, and R. Hardy. 1998. "Meta-analysis of trials comparing antidepressants with active placebos," *Br J Psychiatry*, 172: 227–31.

Moynihan, R. 2008. "Key opinion leaders: Independent experts or drug representatives in disguise?," *BMJ*, 336: 1402–3.

Moynihan, R., I. Heath, and D. Henry. 2002. "Selling sickness: The pharmaceutical industry and disease mongering," *BMJ*, 324: 886–91.

Myers, M. G., J. A. Cairns, and J. Singer. 1987. "The consent form as a possible cause of side effects," *Clin Pharmacol Ther*, 42: 250–3.

Olmsted, J. M. D. 1952. *Claude Bernard and the Experimental Method in Medicine* (H. Schuman: London).

Osler, W. 1948. *Aequanimitas* (The Blakiston Company: Philadelphia, PA).

Pande, A. C., J. G. Crockatt, C. A. Janney, J. L. Werth, and G. Tsaroucha. 2000. "Gabapentin in bipolar disorder: A placebo-controlled trial of adjunctive therapy. Gabapentin Bipolar Disorder Study Group," *Bipolar Disord*, 2: 249–55.

Parascandola, M. 2004. "Skepticism, statistical methods, and the cigarette: A historical analysis of a methodological debate," *Perspect Biol Med*, 47: 244–61.

Parker, G., L. Tully, A. Olley, and D. Hadzi-Pavlovic. 2006. "SSRIs as mood stabilizers for Bipolar II Disorder? A proof of concept study," *J Affect Disord*, 92: 205–14.

Patsopoulos, N. A., J. P. Ioannidis, and A. A. Analatos. 2006. "Origin and funding of the most frequently cited papers in medicine: Database analysis," *BMJ*, 332: 1061–4.

Peirce, C. 1958a. "The fixation of belief," in P. Weiner (ed.), *Selected Writings* (Dover Publications: New York), pp. 91–112.

1958b. *Selected Works* (Dover: New York).

Phelps, J. R., and S. N. Ghaemi. 2006. "Improving the diagnosis of bipolar disorder: Predictive value of screening tests," *J Affect Disord*, 92: 141–8.

Pickering, G. W. 1949. "The place of the experimental method in medicine," *Proc R Soc Med*, 42: 229–34.

Poe, E. A. 1845. *Graham's Magazine*.

Pollard, P., and Richardson, J. T. 1987. "On the probability of making Type I errors," *Psychol. Bull*, 102: 159–63.

Popper, K. 1959. *The Logic of Scientific Discovery* (Basic Books: New York).

Porter, R. 1997. *The Greatest Benefit to Mankind: A Medical History of Humanity* (Norton: New York).

Posternak, M. A., and M. Zimmerman. 2003. "How accurate are patients in reporting their antidepressant treatment history?," *J Affect Disord*, 75: 115–24.

Prentice, R. L., R. D. Langer, M. L. Stefanick, et al. 2006. "Combined analysis of Women's Health Initiative observational and clinical trial data on postmenopausal hormone treatment and cardiovascular disease," *Am J Epidemiol*, 163: 589–99.

Roberts, L. W., T. D. Warner, J. L. Brody, et al. 2002. "Patient and psychiatrist ratings of hypothetical schizophrenia research protocols: Assessment of harm potential and factors influencing participation decisions," *Am J Psychiatry*, 159: 573–84.

Robin, E. D. 1985. "The cult of the Swan-Ganz catheter: Overuse and abuse of pulmonary flow catheters," *Ann Intern Med*, 103: 445–9.

Robins, E., and S. B. Guze. 1970. "Establishment of diagnostic validity in psychiatric illness: Its application to schizophrenia," *Am J Psychiatry*, 126: 983–7.

Rosner, G. L., W. Stadler, and M. J. Ratain. 2002. "Randomized discontinuation design: Application to cytostatic antineoplastic agents," *J Clin Oncol*, 20: 4478–84.

Rothman, K. J., and S. Greenland. 1998. *Modern Epidemiology* (Lippincott-Raven: Philadelphia).

Rush, A. J., M. H. Trivedi, S. R. Wisniewski, et al. 2006. "Acute and longer-term outcomes in depressed outpatients requiring one or several treatment steps: A STAR*D report," *Am J Psychiatry*, 163: 1905–17.

Rush, A. J., M. H. Trivedi, S. R. Wisniewski, et al. 2006. "Bupropion-SR, sertraline, or venlafaxine-XR after failure of SSRIs for depression," *N Engl J Med*, 354: 1231–42.

Ruskin, J. N. 1989. "The cardiac arrhythmia suppression trial (CAST)," *N Engl J Med*, 321: 386–8.

Rutherford, B. R., S. Mori, J. R. Sneed, M. A. Pimontel, and S. P. Roose. 2012. "Contribution of spontaneous improvement to placebo response in depression: A meta-analytic review," *J Psychiatr Res*, 46: 697–702. https://doi.org/10.1016/j.jpsychires.2012.02.008.

Sachs, G. S., F. Grossman, S. N. Ghaemi, A. Okamoto, and C. L. Bowden. 2002. "Combination of a mood stabilizer with risperidone or haloperidol for treatment of acute mania: A double-blind, placebo-controlled comparison of efficacy and safety," *Am J Psychiatry*, 159: 1146–54.

Sachs, G. S., A. A. Nierenberg, J. R. Calabrese, et al. 2007. "Effectiveness of adjunctive antidepressant treatment for bipolar depression," *N Engl J Med*, 356: 1711–22.

Sackett, D. L., S. Strauss, W. S. Richardson, W. Rosenberg, and R. B. Haynes. 2000. *Evidence Based Medicine* (Churchill Livingstone: London).

Salsburg, D. 2001. *The Lady Tasting Tea: How Statistics Revolutionized Science in the Twentieth Century* (W H Freeman and Company: New York).

Schick, E. C., Jr., C. S. Liang, F. A. Heupler, Jr., et al. 1982. "Randomized withdrawal from nifedipine: Placebo-controlled study in patients with coronary artery spasm," *Am Heart J*, 104: 690–7.

Selker, H. P., K. A. Oye, H. G. Eichler, et al. 2013. "A proposal for integrated efficacy-to-effectiveness (E2E) clinical trials," *Clin Pharmacol Ther*, 95: 147–53.

Sharma, M. R., W. M. Stadler, and M. J. Ratain. 2011. "Randomized phase II trials: A long-term investment with promising returns," *J Natl Cancer Inst*, 103: 1093–100.

Shepherd, M. 1993. "The placebo: From specificity to the non-specific and back," *Psychol Med*, 23: 569–78.

Silberman, E. K., and D. A. Snyderman. 1997. "Research without external funding in North American psychiatry," *Am J Psychiatry*, 154: 1159–60.

Silverman, WA. 1998. *Where's the Evidence? Debates in Modern Medicine* (Oxford University Press: New York).

Sleight, P. 2000. "Debate: Subgroup analyses in clinical trials: fun to look at – but don't believe them!" *Curr Control Trials Cardiovasc Med*, 1: 25–7.

Smith, G. C, S., and J. P. Pell. 2003. "Parachute use to prevent death and major trauma related to gravitational challenge: Systematic review of randomized controlled trials," *BMJ*, 327: 1459–61.

Soldani, F., S. N. Ghaemi, and R. Baldessarini. 2005. "Research methods in psychiatric treatment studies: Critique and proposals," *Acta Psychiatr Scand*, 112: 1–3.

Sox, H. C., and D. Rennie. 2006. "Research misconduct, retraction, and cleansing the medical literature: Lessons from the Poehlman case," *Ann Intern Med*, 144: 609–13.

Sprock, J. 1988. "Classification of schizoaffective disorder," *Compr. Psychiatry*, 29: 55–71.

Stahl, S. M. 2002. "Antipsychotic polypharmacy: Evidence based or eminence based?" *Acta Psychiatr Scand*, 106: 321–2.

2005. *Essential Psychopharmacology* (Cambridge University Press: Cambridge UK).

Stigler, S. M. 1986. *The History of Statistics: The Measurement of Uncertainty before 1900* (Harvard University Press: Cambridge, MA).

Suppes, T., E. Vieta, S. Liu, M. Brecher, and B. Paulsson. 2009. "Maintenance treatment for patients with bipolar I disorder: Results from a North American study of quetiapine in combination with lithium or divalproex (trial 127)," *Am J Psychiatry*, 166: 476–88.

Tatsioni, A., N. G. Bonitsis, and J. P. Ioannidis. 2007. "Persistence of contradicted claims in the literature," *JAMA*, 298: 2517–26.

Turner, E. H., A. M. Matthews, E. Linardatos, R. A. Tell, and R. Rosenthal. 2008. "Selective publication of antidepressant trials and its influence on apparent efficacy," *N Engl J Med*, 358: 252–60.

Vieta, E., T. Suppes, I. Eggens, et al. 2008. "Efficacy and safety of quetiapine in combination with lithium or divalproex for maintenance of patients with bipolar I disorder (international trial 126)," *J Affect Disord*, 109: 251–63.

Wang, R., S. W. Lagakos, J. H. Ware, D. J. Hunter, and J. M. Drazen. 2007. "Statistics in medicine–reporting of subgroup analyses in clinical trials," *N Engl J Med*, 357: 2189–94.

Weisler, R. H., W. A. Nolen, A. Neijber, A. Hellqvist, and B. Paulsson. 2011. "Continuation of quetiapine versus switching to placebo or lithium for maintenance treatment of bipolar i disorder (trial 144: A randomized controlled study)," *J Clin Psychiatry*, 72: 1452–64. http://dx.doi.org/10.4088/JCP.11m06878.

Yastrubetskaya, O., E. Chiu, and S. O'Connell. 1997. "Is good clinical research practice for clinical trials good clinical practice?" *Int J Geriatr Psychiatry*, 12: 227–31.

Zimmerman, M., J. I. Mattia, and M. A. Posternak. 2002. "Are subjects in pharmacological treatment trials of depression representative of patients in routine clinical practice?" *Am J Psychiatry*, 159: 469–73.

Index